The *Source* for Children with Cochlear Implants

David J. Ertmer, Ph.D.

Content Areas:	Cochlear implant technology
	Communication intervention
Ages:	Birth – Adolescence

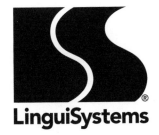

LinguiSystems

LinguiSystems, Inc.
3100 4th Ave
East Moline, Il 61265

800-776-4332

FAX: 800-577-4555
E-mail: service@linguisystems.com
Web: linguisystems.com

Printed in the U.S.A.
ISBN 10: 0-7606-0548-3
ISBN 13: 978-0-7606-0548-6

About the Author

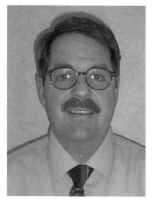 **David J. Ertmer**, Ph.D., is an associate professor in Audiology and Speech Sciences at Purdue University, West Lafayette, Indiana. He received a B.S. from Marquette University, a M.S. from the University of Wisconsin – Milwaukee, and a Ph.D. from Purdue University, all in the field of Communication Disorders. His clinical career includes 17 years as a school speech pathologist in Wisconsin and Colorado. Currently, he teaches courses in aural rehabilitation and clinical methods, and conducts research in early speech and language development in young children with hearing loss. David and his wife Peg, an associate professor in Educational Technology at Purdue University, have four children. He is also the author of *Contrasts for Auditory & Speech Training (CAST)*.

Dedication

This book is respectfully dedicated to three groups of people: the children with hearing loss whom I have known through the years, their families, and their teachers. Your determination and zest for life have been both educational and inspirational.

Acknowledgments

I am very appreciative of the many colleagues who have given invaluable suggestions and feedback as this book was being written. These generous individuals include Linda Charlebois, Kristen Corbett, Kristi Grohne, Laura Kretschmer, Richard Kretschmer, Jeannette Leonard, Suneeti Nathani, Peggy Nelson, Ronnie Wilbur, and Michelle Wilkins. Thanks also to Karen Stontz for her expertise and patience as editor for this project.

Edited by Karen Stontz
Page Layout by Christine Buysse
Cover Art and Illustrations by Margaret Warner
Cover Design by Mike Paustian

Table of Contents

Table of Contents

Preface

These are truly exciting times for deaf children, their families, and professionals in the fields of communication disorders and education. Nearly 15 years of rigorous research has shown that consistent use of a cochlear implant (CI) can lead to greatly improved auditory perception, closer-to-normal rates of language development, and increased opportunities for integration in regular classrooms (ASHA 2004). The advent of Universal Newborn Hearing Screening (UNHS) and recent reductions in the age criterion for implantation (currently 12 months) have also made it possible for deaf toddlers to begin to hear during a crucial period for language development. In short, today—as never before—deaf children have the potential to become fully participating members of society at large.

Although there are good reasons to be optimistic about the future for children with cochlear implants, two important realities must be kept in mind. First, research has shown that there is considerable variability in the oral communication abilities of children with CIs (See Kirk 2000 for review). That is, children will differ in the rates at which they develop listening, speech, and oral language skills after implantation. Secondly, advances in these areas result from a combination of CI use and clinical intervention. It has become clear that the implant, by itself, does not guarantee the development of adequate spoken language ability; effective intervention programs are needed to facilitate auditory and oral skill development. Stated another way, the quality of the services provided by speech-language pathologists, audiologists, and educators of children with hearing loss can make a significant difference in the functional benefits that children receive from their implants. As increasing numbers of children with CIs receive services through regular education agencies, there is a pressing need to disseminate information about the implant itself and about intervention procedures that are designed to optimize auditory-oral learning after implantation.

Cochlear implantation is a relatively new approach to treating deafness in children. Professionals who graduated before 1990 did not routinely have access to courses in cochlear implant technology or specialized interventions for children who have CIs. Those who graduated more recently may not have selected CI-related courses as electives, or attended programs that offered such courses. *The Source for Children with Cochlear Implants* has two main purposes: to serve as a comprehensive guide to the cochlear implant field for practicing professionals and to act as an introductory textbook for students in the field of communication disorders. It was also designed to be a source of materials and clinical ideas for a wide age range of children. To this end, a variety of informal assessment tools and forms can be photocopied, and lists of recommended readings and Internet resources are provided for clinicians and parents alike.

I sincerely hope that you will find *The Source for Children with Cochlear Implants* to be an informative and practical resource as you help children reach their potentials as communicators, students, and citizens.

DJE

References

Cochlear Implants (2004). Technical report. Washington, D.C.: American Speech-Language-Hearing Association.

Kirk, K. I. (2000). Challenges in the clinical investigation of cochlear implant outcomes. In J. Niparko, K. I. Kirk, N. Mellon, A. Robbins, D. Tucci, and B. Wilson (Eds.), *Cochlear Implants: Principles and Practice* (pp. 225-259). Philadelphia: Lippincott Williams & Wilkins, Inc.

Introduction to Part 1
Cochlear Implant Technology and Follow-up Services

The first five chapters of this book provide a wide-ranging tour of cochlear implant (CI) technology, an overview of the professional responsibilities of implant team members, practical considerations for selecting a mode of communication for children with implants, and recommendations for taking care of this incredible electronic device.

The tour begins with an account of the surprisingly long history of efforts to stimulate hearing through electrical stimulation. From crude electric shocks delivered to the external ear (Don't try this at home!) to the small ear-level, multi-channel implants of today, you will gain an increased appreciation of the insightful advancements made by early and modern developers alike. Chapter 1 also provides a basic description of the components and the functions of currently available CIs. This information describes how implants work, how they differ from hearing aids, and how electrical stimulation can convey essential information about the speech signal.

Chapter 2 walks you through the issues that must be considered as parents and professionals consider whether a cochlear implant is the right choice for a child. Candidacy criterion and pre-implantation evaluations are discussed in detail to give a clear picture of the decision-making process.

Chapter 3 allows you to "look over the shoulders" of the surgeon and the audiologist as the implant is placed during a two-hour operation, as the CI is activated for the first time, and as parents observe their child's first response to sound via the implant. Although most of you will not be actively involved in these situations, this chapter will help you appreciate the exacting efforts needed to make sure the implant is properly placed and optimally mapped.

In addition to deciding to provide an implant, parents of very young children may still be attempting to choose the communication modality that best suits their child and family. Chapter 4 details the pros and cons of Oral, Total Communication, Cued Speech, and American Sign Language for children with CIs. A variety of educational options are also considered.

Finally, to be effective, the implant must work properly every day. Chapter 5 leads parents and clinicians through essential checks to ensure that the implant is maintained in good working condition.

Cochlear Implant Technology

What Is a Cochlear Implant?

Cochlear implants (CIs) are electronic devices that increase hearing sensitivity in individuals who receive limited benefit from hearing aids. These surgically implanted sensory aids improve hearing by circumventing damaged receptor cells in the cochlea and providing electrical stimulation directly to the auditory nerve. Cochlear implants typically enable deaf children and adults to make substantial improvements in their speech detection and perception abilities.

How Do Cochlear Implants Differ from Hearing Aids?

Hearing Aids (HAs) are the most commonly prescribed and successfully used technology for overcoming mild, moderate, and severe hearing losses. However, HAs typically provide insufficient access to speech at conversational intensity levels for children and adults with profound hearing losses (i.e., pure-tone averages greater than 90 dB HL). Multi-channel cochlear implants are viable alternatives to HAs for these individuals because they provide relatively greater increases in hearing sensitivity and improved potential for oral communication.

There are two basic differences in the ways that HAs and CIs increase hearing sensitivity. First, the output of HAs (whether analog or digital) is an amplified (louder) acoustic signal. In contrast, the output of a CI is an electrical signal. The second difference has to do with the "paths" these signals take. The amplified acoustic signal from a hearing aid follows the normal path through the outer, middle, and inner ear. For individuals with sensorineural hearing loss, however, important features of the signal remain inaudible despite amplification because receptor cells in the inner ear are damaged or missing. The impact of this damage is usually most severe in the high frequencies. The electrical CI signal, on the other hand, bypasses both the middle ear and the damaged receptor cells in the cochlea to stimulate the auditory nerve directly. Electrical stimulation of the auditory nerve results in improved hearing sensitivity across a wide range of frequencies (approximately 250–7000 Hz) for most implant users. In summary, HAs enable hard-of-hearing individuals to take advantage of their residual hearing by increasing the "loudness" of the auditory signal. CIs enable individuals with little or no residual hearing capacity to hear by stimulating the auditory nerve directly.

A Brief History of Cochlear Implant Technology

Although cochlear implants first became commercially available in the 1970s, the possibility of using electricity to stimulate hearing has been investigated for more than two centuries. The following is a condensed account of some of the major events that led to the sophisticated implant technology of today. Readers who would like to learn more about this topic are encouraged to consult House (1995), Clark (1997), and Niparko and Wilson (2000).

Late 1700s	Allessandro Volta applies electrical current to a circuit formed by inserting a rounded metallic probe in each of his ears. He reports hearing a loud boom and a series of crackling sounds similar to those produced by a thick, boiling soup. Fearing damage to his brain, Volta prudently decides not to repeat the experiment.
1800s	Attempts to stimulate hearing using direct electrical current yield unsatisfactory results. Brenner (1868) investigates the effects of polarity, rate, and intensity of electrical stimulus and electrode placement on hearing stimulation. He finds that negative polarity and the placement of an electrode outside of the ear improve hearing sensations.
1930–1940s	Improved understanding of hearing physiology leads to the conclusion that the treatment of deafness will require localized stimulation of the auditory nerve, rather than widespread stimulation of the hearing mechanism.
1950s	Two Frenchmen, Djourno and Eyries (1957), place an electrical wire on the auditory nerve of a deaf man during surgery. The patient reports perceiving sounds resembling crickets and roulette wheels. Interest increases for the development of an implantable device to treat deafness.

1960s	Dr. William F. House and colleagues surgically implant several deaf adult volunteers with single channel cochlear implant prototypes. Although the devices function well, they are explanted due to bio-incompatibility problems with the insulating materials. A percutaneous (through the skin) connection is developed for the 3M/House single-channel implant. The connection directly links the internal receiver/stimulator to the external sound processor. Testing is conducted only during brief laboratory sessions because of concern for damaging remaining neural tissue.
1970s	House and colleagues develop the first wearable single-channel implant for everyday use. An adult recipient reports improved hearing for a variety of sounds. An external speech processor for the single-channel 3M/House implant is marketed commercially (1972). The "First International Conference on the Electrical Stimulation of the Auditory Nerve as a Treatment for Sensorineural Deafness in Man" is held at the University of California–San Francisco (1974). The 3M/House single-channel cochlear implant is modified to include internal and external magnets. The magnets hold the external components in place behind the ear to permit transcutaneous (across the skin) transmission of the processed signal via FM radio waves (1975). Extensive research into the capabilities of the 3M/House single-channel implant system verifies hearing benefits for deaf adults (Bilger et al. 1977). This report also recommends the development of multi-channel cochlear implants to take advantage of the tonotopic organization of the cochlea.
1980s	The 3M/House single-channel cochlear implant becomes the first device approved by the U.S. Food and Drug Administration (FDA) to replace a human sense (1984). Children begin to receive single-channel cochlear implants. Implant criteria is lowered from 18 to 2 years of age throughout the decade. The Nucleus 22-electrode, multi-channel cochlear implant receives FDA approval for use in postlingually deafened adults (1985).

continued on next page

The Source for Children with Cochlear Implants   13

1990s	The Nucleus 22-cochlear implant is approved for children two years and older. A variety of electrode configurations and speech processing strategies are developed by cochlear implant manufacturers. The Clarion cochlear implant system receives FDA approval for adults (1996) and for children (1997). The Nucleus cochlear implant is approved for use with adults who have severe hearing impairments. Ear-level speech processors become available (1999).
2000– present	The MED-EL Combi 40+ cochlear implant system receives FDA approval in the United States (2001). The system, widely used throughout Europe, includes an ear-level speech processor. Clarion Corporation introduces an in-the-ear microphone for use with telephones and headphones (2002). Research into bilateral implantation is begun. Age criterion for children is lowered to 12 months for the Clarion, Nucleus, and MED-EL devices. To date, more than 60,000 people have received cochlear implants worldwide. More than 14,000 of these have been implanted in the United States. Approximately half of all implant users are children.

What Are the Components of a Cochlear Implant?

CIs have internal and external components. The internal parts consist of a receiver/stimulator unit, electrode lead cables, and a group of electrodes called an *array*. These can be seen in the lower left-hand portion of Figure 1.1. The main external components are a power source (batteries), a microphone, an FM radio transmitter, and a speech processor. The radio transmitter is held in place over the internal receiver/stimulator by magnets. The radio transmitters are the disk-like objects in the upper and lower-right implant systems shown in Figure 1.1. Speech processors can be worn in a variety of places on the body and are connected to the external transmitter by electrical cables. For example, very young children may wear their speech processors in harnesses on their backs so that they are out of the way. Older children may wear their processors in a pouch on the chest, stomach, or under the arm. Newly developed, smaller processors are worn at ear-level or clipped to clothing. Microphones may be part of the transmitter, part of the speech processor unit, or independent of these components, depending on the manufacturer. Figure 1.1 shows the Nucleus SPrint body-worn speech processor (top) and the Nucleus ESPrit 3G ear-level implant system (lower right).

Figure 1.1: Isolated Components of a Nucleus ESPrit 3G Cochlear Implant

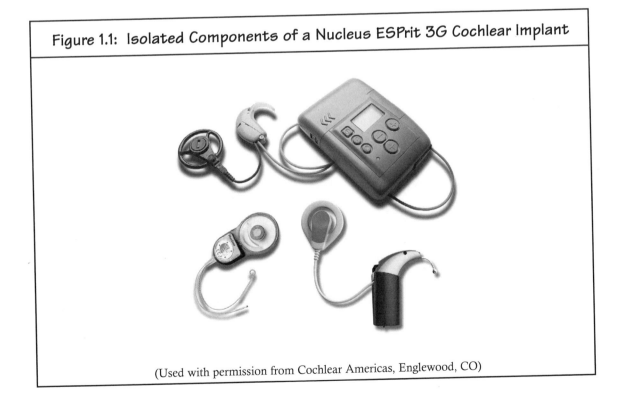

(Used with permission from Cochlear Americas, Englewood, CO)

As the illustration below shows, the receiver/stimulator unit is positioned just under the skin in a surgically hollowed-out portion of the temporal bone. The electrode lead cable winds from the receiver/stimulator through a channel drilled from the temporal bone to the middle ear. The electrode array is inserted into the cochlea through the round window and extended toward the apex of the cochlea, running along the basilar membrane in the scala tympani. The external and internal components of the Nucleus ESPrit 3G cochlear implant system are shown in place in Figure 1.2.

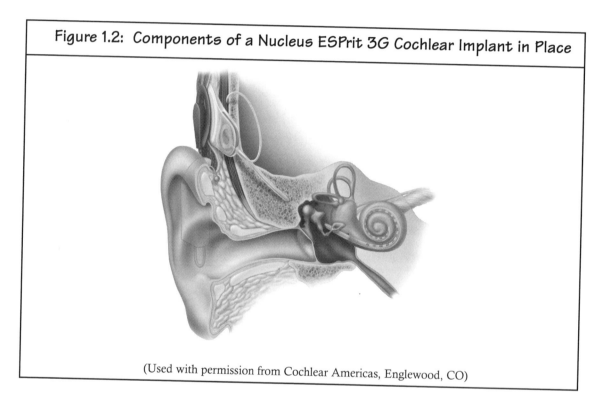

Figure 1.2: Components of a Nucleus ESPrit 3G Cochlear Implant in Place

(Used with permission from Cochlear Americas, Englewood, CO)

How Does a Cochlear Implant Work?

Cochlear implants increase hearing sensitivity by transforming acoustic energy into an electrical signal that can be introduced to the nervous system and interpreted by the brain. The following is a basic description of ways in which sound is transformed and processed by multi-channel CIs. For a more in-depth discussion of the topic, see Wilson (1993, 2000).

1. The microphone detects sound and converts it into an electrical signal.

2. The electrical signal is passed to the speech processor via cables where it is digitized and manipulated according to the selected speech processing strategy.

3. The modified electronic signal or "code" leaves the speech processor and is passed to an external FM radio transmitter held in place over the internal receiver/stimulator by magnets. The transmitter converts the electronic code to a radio wave that is broadcast across the skin to the internal receiver/stimulator.

4. The internal receiver/stimulator receives the FM signal and converts it into an electronic code.   This code determines how the individual electrodes or groups of electrodes (called *channels*) within the cochlea are turned on and off. The precise manner in which the electrodes are activated is determined by the implant audiologist.

Why Do Multi-Channel Cochlear Implants Work?

Cochlear implants convey vital information about the frequency, intensity, and timing of speech and environmental sounds. The tonotopic organization of the cochlea and the auditory nerve provides the basis for representing the frequencies of speech and environmental sounds to the central nervous system.

In the normal ear, low frequency sounds are perceived when the sensory cells close to the apex of the cochlea are stimulated. Progressively higher frequencies are perceived as sensory cells toward the base of the cochlea are stimulated. The implant takes advantage of this natural arrangement to convey frequency information to the auditory nerve by activating electrodes at different locations along the basilar membrane (see the electrode array in Figure 1.2).

In the implanted ear, low frequency sounds are represented by activating electrodes near the tip of the array because these electrodes are the closest to the apex of the cochlea. Progressively higher frequency sounds are represented by activating electrodes positioned toward the base of the cochlea. Most speech sounds are well within the frequency representation capacity of multi-channel CIs.

CIs also provide information about the intensity and timing of speech and environmental sounds. Sound intensity (perceived as loudness) is represented by the amount of voltage emitted by the electrodes. Loud sounds are associated with higher voltage levels and soft sounds with lower voltage levels. Timing information (e.g., the durations of speech sounds, rate of formant transitions, pauses) is conveyed by the rate at which individual or groups of electrodes are turned on and off. Recently-developed microcomputers permit electrodes to be turned on and off at very high rates (e.g., up to 91,000 pulses per second in the Clarion CII Bionic ear system). Thus, the phonetic characteristics of the acoustic speech signal (frequency, intensity, and timing) are preserved in the electrical signal provided by multi-channel cochlear implants.

What Are the Main Differences Between Cochlear Implant Models?

There are three major manufacturers of multi-channel cochlear implants available in the United States: Advanced Bionics (Sylmar, CA), Cochlear Americas (Englewood, CO), and MED-EL Corporation (Durham, NC). Although each manufacturer produces several models of implants and each model has distinctive features, the external and internal components of all cochlear implants perform the same basic functions described above. Differences between implants are most often found in speech processing strategies, processing speed, number of electrodes, electrode arrays, types of stimulation, positions of the microphone, locations of ground electrodes, and accessories. Pictures of the Advanced Bionics and MED-EL implant systems can be seen on the next page.

Figure 1.3a: Body-Worn Clarion Platinum Sound Processor and Transmitter

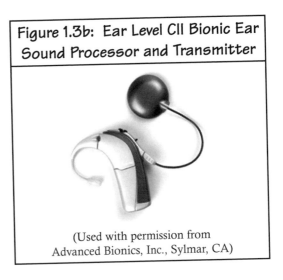

(Used with permission from Advanced Bionics, Inc., Sylmar, CA)

Figure 1.3b: Ear Level CII Bionic Ear Sound Processor and Transmitter

(Used with permission from Advanced Bionics, Inc., Sylmar, CA)

Figure 1.3c: Clarion Receiver/Stimulator Unit

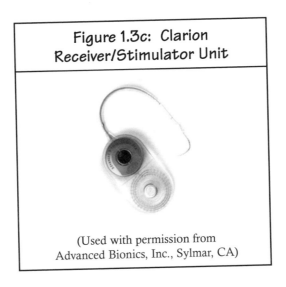

(Used with permission from Advanced Bionics, Inc., Sylmar, CA)

Figure 1.4: External Components of the MED-EL Tempo Ear-Level Cochlear Implant

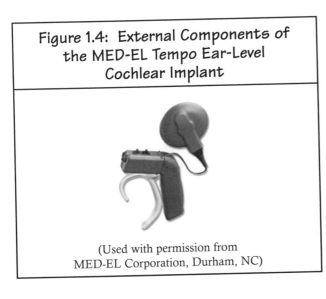

(Used with permission from MED-EL Corporation, Durham, NC)

Figure 1.5: External Components of the MED-EL Tempo "Baby Bte" Speech Processor

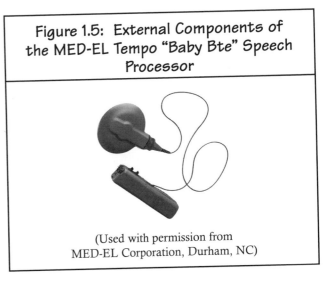

(Used with permission from MED-EL Corporation, Durham, NC)

What Are Speech Processing Strategies?

There are a variety of ways in which implant electrodes can be activated to stimulate the auditory nerve. These activation options are known as *speech processing strategies*. Each strategy employs digital speech processors to transform the signal from the implant microphone into frequency bands that correspond to electrodes or groups of electrodes (channels) within the implant array. Moore and Teagle (2002) point out that there are three main categories of speech processing strategies: those designed to represent mainly the frequency components of speech (e.g., F0/F1/F2, MultiPeak, Spectral Peak); those that emphasize timing characteristics (e.g., Compressed Analog, Simultaneous Analog Samplers, Continuous Interleaved Sampling); and those that highlight both frequency and timing (e.g., Advanced Combination Encoder, n of m strategies). The number of electrodes, number of channels, and the rate in which electrodes are "fired" also vary across implant models. The speech processing strategies of the Nucleus devices can be found in Table 1.1 (page 21), and strategies for the Advanced Bionics and MED-EL devices can be found in Table 1.2 (page 22). For additional information on speech processing strategies, please refer to Moore and Teagle (2002) and Wilson (1993, 2000). Information on speech processing can also be found in the owner's manual and teacher's guide that each manufacturer provides.

Although advances in implant technology and speech processing strategies hold great promise for children with severe to profound hearing losses, the risks and benefits of implantation must be considered for each potential recipient. This careful assessment is the responsibility of the members of the cochlear implant team. The next chapter reviews the roles of team members in determining candidacy for implantation, providing the implant, and offering follow-up services.

Chapter 1: Cochlear Implant Technology

Table 1.1: Features and Speech Processing Strategies for Nucleus Cochlear Implants

Internal Device	Year of Introduction	External Hardware "Trade Name"	Speech Processing Strategy	Bands of Information Delivered to the Patient
Nucleus CI-22	1983	Wearable Speech Processor (WSP)	F0 F2	2
Nucleus Mini CI-22	1987 1989 1994 2000 2004	WSP Mini Speech Processor (MSP) SPECTRA-22 ESPrit – ear level 3G – 22	F0 F1 F2 MPEAK or Multipeak Spectral Peak or SPEAK SPEAK SPEAK	3 4 – 5 6 – 10 average 20 maximum (6 – 10/20) 6 – 10/20 6 – 10/20
Nucleus CI-24 M	1996 1997	SPRINT – BODY WORN ESPrit-22 ear level	SPEAK CIS ACE SPEAK	6 – 10/22 6 – 12 Dynamic /n of m 6 – 10/22
Nucleus CI-24 K	2000	SPRINT – body worn ESPrit – ear level	SPEAK CIS ACE SPEAK	6 – 10/22 6 – 12 Dynamic /n of m 6 – 10/22
Nucleus 24 Contour	1999	SPRINT – body worn ESPrit – ear level	SPEAK CIS ACE SPEAK CIS ACE	6 – 10/22 6 – 12 Dynamic /n of m 6 6 - 12 8/20

Table 1.2: Features and Speech Processing Strategies for Advanced Bionics and MED-EL Cochlear Implants

Manufacturer	Internal Device	Year of Introduction	External Hardware	Speech Processing Strategy	Number of Bands of Information Delivered to the Patient
Advanced Bionics	Spiral electrode	1991	1.0 processor	CIS	8
		1995	1.2 processor	CIS	8
		1997	S-Series	CIS	8
		1999	Platinum Series	CIS, MPS, SAS	8
	Hi FOCUS electrode array	2000	Platinum BTE	CIS, MPS, SAS	8
	CII – Bionic Ear receiver	2001	Platinum Series & CII BTE	CIS, MPS, SAS, HiResolution	16 maximum
		2003	HiRes Auria	HiResolution	16 maximum
MED-EL	Combi 40+	1996	CIS Pro – body worn	CIS	12
	Combi 40+ S (Compressed array for partial ossification)	1997	CIS Pro – body worn	CIS	12
					Dynamic/n of m
	Combi 40+ GB (Split array for complete ossification)	1998	Tempo+ – BTE	CIS	12
				CIS+	Dynamic/n of m

References

Clark, G. (1997). Historical perspectives. In G. Clark, R. Cowan, and R. Dowell (Eds.), *Cochlear implantation for infants and children* (pp. 9 - 28). San Diego, CA: Singular.

House, W. F. (1995). *Cochlear implants: My perspective.* Newport Beach, CA: AllHear, Inc.

Moore, J. A. and Teagle, H. F. B. (2002). An introduction to cochlear implant technology, activation, and programming. *Language, Speech, and Hearing Services in Schools*, 33, 153-161.

Niparko, J. and Wilson, B. (2000). History of cochlear implants. In J. Niparko, K. I. Kirk, N. Mellon, A. Robbins, D. Tucci, and B. Wilson (Eds.), *Cochlear implants principles and practices* (pp. 103-108). Philadelphia: Lippincott Williams & Wilkins, Inc.

Wilson, B. (1993). Signal processing. In R. Tyler (Ed.), *Cochlear implants: Audiological foundations* (pp. 35-86). San Diego, CA: Singular.

Wilson, B. (2000). Cochlear implant technology. In J. Niparko, K. Kirk, N. Mellon, A. Robbins, D. Tucci, and B. Wilson (Eds.), *Cochlear implants: Principles & practices* (pp. 109-118). Philadelphia: Lippincott Williams & Wilkins, Inc.

The Cochlear Implant
Decision-Making Process

As mentioned in Chapter 1, cochlear implants are not appropriate for everyone with a hearing loss. In most cases, less-expensive and less-invasive hearing aids continue to be the best choice for children with mild, moderate, or severe hearing losses. However, the cautious implantation criteria of the 1980s and early 1990s have gradually expanded to include younger children and children with more residual hearing. This loosening of candidacy requirements has occurred for two main

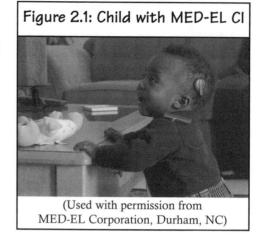

Figure 2.1: Child with MED-EL CI

(Used with permission from
MED-EL Corporation, Durham, NC)

reasons. First, hearing sensitivity criteria have been lowered as the performances of some deaf children have approximated or exceeded that of children with better residual hearing who use hearing aids. Although implanted children vary in the amount of benefit received from a CI, a large percentage show oral communication gains beyond what could reasonably be expected with continued use of hearing aids. Secondly, age requirements have decreased as the advantages of a younger age-at-implantation have become apparent (e.g., Ertmer and Mellon 2001, Kirk et al. 2002, Waltzman and Cohen 1998). Lower age criteria reflect the belief that implantation during the first two years of life may lead to more efficient acquisition of oral communication skills than implantation later in life.

General criteria for cochlear implantation in the United States and Canada require that children be 12 months of age or older; have bilateral, profound hearing impairments (i.e., better-ear, three-frequency pure-tone average of 90 dB HL or greater); wear well-fitted hearing aids for three to six months; and show little or no benefit from amplification. In extenuating situations, such as incidents of ossification (bony growth) in the cochlea, children younger than 12 months have also received cochlear implants. In some cases, children who have severe hearing losses (i.e., PTAs between 70–90 dB HL) with poor aided speech perception ability may also be accepted for implantation.

In addition to these basic requirements, most implant centers complete a variety of health, audiological, psychological, and educational assessments to determine whether a child is an appropriate implant candidate. These assessments are typically completed by family physicians; otologists/Ear, Nose, and Throat (ENT) specialists; radiologists; audiologists; speech-language pathologists, psychologists; and educators of the hearing impaired. The actual size and makeup of the implant team varies from center to center. The following sections describe procedures that are commonly completed during the cochlear implant decision-making process.

Medical and Radiologic Evaluations

The rigors of implant surgery dictate that a physical exam and health history be completed to determine whether the child is in good health, is able to tolerate anesthesia, and is free of active middle ear pathologies (e.g., otitis media). These initial exams are completed by a family physician and the child's otologist.

Several tests are used to examine the physical status of hearing structures. Computed Tomography (CT) scans and Magnetic Resonance Imaging (MRI) provide images of the temporal bone and the inner ear prior to implantation. These procedures enable radiologists and surgeons to determine whether internal, hearing-related structures are properly formed, and whether there is ossification in the cochlea. Cochlear malformations and ossification can limit the number of electrodes that can be inserted into the cochlea. A modified surgical approach may be necessary for children with these concerns. In rare cases, children's cochleae may be absent or so poorly developed that implantation is not possible.

Promontory Stimulation is used to check the responsiveness of the auditory nerve to electrical stimulation. This procedure involves sending an electrical current through the round window of the cochlea and measuring neural responses through electrodes placed around the cranium. Cochlear implantation is contraindicated for individuals who have no responses to Promontory Stimulation. For example, tumors in retro-cochlear auditory pathways can inhibit the transmission of the hearing sensations to the central nervous system. In such cases, stimulation of the auditory nerve at the level of the cochlea would not facilitate improved hearing. Patients with auditory nerve pathologies may be candidates for an Auditory Brainstem Implant (ABI). ABIs involve placing stimulating electrodes in or on the brainstem rather than in the cochlea (Tucci and Niparko 2000).

Audiologic Evaluations

Assessing Hearing Sensitivity

In general, the age of the child determines what kinds of tests are used to measure pre-implant hearing ability. For children less than six months, Auditory Brainstem Response (ABR) testing and Steady State Evoked Potentials (SSEP) provide objective estimates of hearing thresholds without requiring active participation by the child. In addition, Otoacoustic Emissions (OAE) testing can be helpful in determining whether the hearing loss is cochlear in origin.

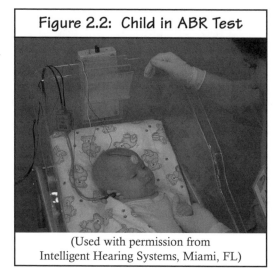

Figure 2.2: Child in ABR Test

(Used with permission from Intelligent Hearing Systems, Miami, FL)

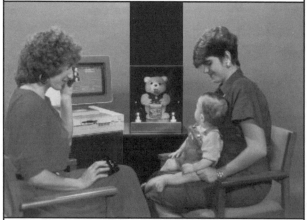

Figure 2.3: Child in VRA Session

(Used with permission from Intelligent Hearing Systems, Miami, FL)

Children between six months and four years are often capable, to varying degrees, of participating in behavioral hearing testing through Visually Reinforced Audiometry (VRA). Using operant conditioning principles, children are taught to associate a visual reinforcer (e.g., a lit-up, moving toy figure) with presentations of an auditory signal (pure tones, warble tones, or speech). Auditory detection is presumed when the child turns to look for the visual reinforcer immediately after the auditory signal is presented. These procedures are used before and after HAs have been fitted to document unaided and aided hearing levels.

Children older than four years are able to participate in behavioral and play audiometry to determine aided and unaided hearing sensitivity levels. They demonstrate detection of tones and speech by raising their hands, placing pegs in a pegboard, or stacking blocks whenever they hear a stimulus. Behavioral measures are completed several times before surgery to ensure a consistent estimate of hearing sensitivity and to confirm ABR, SSEP, and OAE results. Tympanometry is also conducted multiple times prior to implant surgery to aid in detecting middle ear pathologies such as otitis media. Medications and/or ventilation tubes are prescribed, as needed, to clear up middle ear problems prior to surgery.

A hearing aid trial is required prior to cochlear implantation. Many young deaf children need special training to respond to sound during this time. Two simple techniques can make sound more salient to children who have new hearing aids. First, parents and clinicians can provide "listening models" by making their own responses to sound more overt. For example, a mother may act startled and point to her ear while saying "I hear that" whenever the telephone rings, someone speaks loudly, or a dog barks. Secondly, praise and edible rewards (i.e., cereal bits) can be used to reinforce the child whenever he indicates that he has heard something. Listening should be emphasized throughout the day so that the child comes to see it as an important and enjoyable experience.

Vibro-tactile aids can also help to make sound more salient for children who are beginning to use hearing aids. Commercially available "tactaids" such as the Tacticulator and the Tactaid-7 (see Figure 2.4) consist of a microphone, a speech processor, and a set of vibrators. The vibrators are typically worn in a pouch on the chest and become activated in the presence of sound. The goal of tactaid use is to help children associate vibrations on the skin with hearing sensations. Parents and interventionists facilitate this connection by using the listening models and behavioral reinforcement procedures described above. Tactaid use is usually decreased as children respond to sound more consistently so that the benefits of amplification can be examined more directly.

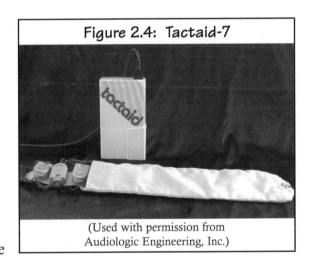

Figure 2.4: Tactaid-7

(Used with permission from Audiologic Engineering, Inc.)

Assessing Speech Perception Ability

In addition to measuring children's ability to detect sound, it is important to estimate how well they perceive speech. Again, the age of the child usually influences the type of assessment. For infants and toddlers, responsiveness to speech is examined during everyday activities. These functional assessments involve observing the child's responses to sound during evaluation sessions and gathering information on responsiveness to sound through parent reports. Questions, such as "Does the child turn when his name is called?" and "Does he recognize the difference between parents' voices?" help to estimate both detection and speech perception abilities. Parental reports of auditory behaviors are also important for verifying behavioral, ABR, and SSEP thresholds and for estimating benefit from hearing aids.

Speech perception testing can be more direct for preschool and school-age children. Closed-set and open-set speech recognition tests are commonly used with children who can maintain attention and have at least a rudimentary vocabulary. In most cases, the stimuli (e.g., isolated vowels, syllables, words, sentences) are presented without any speechreading cues (i.e., auditory-only condition). Speech perception can also be examined when auditory and speechreading cues are available (i.e., Auditory + Visual [A +V] condition). Testing under the latter condition can provide an indication of how well children understand speech in everyday, face-to-face situations.

Closed-set tests require children to identify auditory stimulus items from among sets of choices. For example, the *Children's Vowel Perception Test* (Tyler et al. 1991) contains sets of pictures that represent minimal pair vowel contrasts. The objective of this particular test is to determine whether the child recognizes acoustic cues for vowels with greater than chance accuracy. For example, children are asked to identify "cat" from a set of pictures representing a kite, a coat, a cat, and a cut. Because the chance of guessing the answer correctly is one in four, children's total test scores must be significantly higher than 25% correct to demonstrate closed-set identification ability. In addition to assessing vowel contrasts, closed-set tests can also be used to assess the ability to identify a wide range of auditory stimuli including suprasegmental or timing/intensity patterns such as long vs. short sounds and continuous vs. interrupted sounds (e.g., *The Glendonald Auditory Screening Procedure*, Erber 1982; *The Early Speech Perception Test*, Moog and Geers 1990); and segmental features in words (e.g., *Minimal Pairs Test*, Robbins et al. 1988).

Open-set tests require children to identify spoken words, phrases, or sentences without sets of choices. These procedures usually call for children to listen to a speech stimulus item and then repeat it aloud. Commonly administered open-set word recognition tests include the *Phonetically Balanced Kindergarten Test* (*PB-K*, Haskins 1949) and the *Lexical Neighborhood Test* (Kirk et al. 1995). Sentence recognition tests include the *CID Sentences* (Davis and Silverman 1978) and the *Pediatric Speech Intelligibility Sentence Test* (Jerger et al. 1980). Reviews of a variety of commonly used closed- and open-set tests can be found in Tyler (1993) and Kirk (2000).

In summary, prior to implantation, audiologists determine how well children can detect sound with and without hearing aids, and the degree to which speech has become recognizable and meaningful during the hearing aid trial. This information is essential for ensuring that children undergo cochlear implant surgery only if the auditory outcomes of implantation are expected to exceed those achieved through hearing aid use.

Communication Assessments

Speech-language pathologists participate in the implant decision-making process in several important ways. For children under three years, they provide communication evaluations that focus on the emergence of prelinguistic and early linguistic skills. The former area includes assessment of the frequency and diversity of communication attempts (e.g., use of gestures, facial expressions) and participation in communication opportunities (e.g., getting attention, turn-taking skills). The child's prelinguistic speech can also be examined for canonical syllables (i.e., consonant and vowel combinations with adult-like timing [Lynch et al. 1989]) and for more advanced speech forms such as jargon (syllable strings with varied consonants, vowels, and changing intonation or stress), as well as the diversity of vowel and consonant types (Ertmer and Mellon 2001, Nathani et al. 2002). Increases in the diversity, complexity, and speech-like nature of spontaneous vocalizations, and improved ability to imitate speech sounds can indicate benefit from hearing aids during the trial period.

Comprehension and production of spoken words and the use of word combinations should also be monitored. For young children, these skills are typically assessed through parent reports such as the *Communication Development Inventory* (Fenson et al. 1993) and by observing parent-child interactions during play activities.

For children three years and older, observations of communication ability and responsiveness to sound are often supplemented with formal language tests and samples. Estimates of receptive and expressive vocabulary size and the use of morphological markers are made with tests developed for normally hearing children (e.g., *Peabody Picture Vocabulary Test III*, Dunn et al. 1997) or those standardized for children with hearing loss (e.g., *Grammatical Analysis of Elicited Language*, Moog et al. 1983). To be valid, formal language tests and language samples must be conducted in the child's mode of communication (e.g., Oral Communication, Simultaneous Communication, American Sign Language). Qualified interpreters are used when clinicians are not fluent in the child's modality. Communication modalities will be discussed in Chapter 4.

For school-age children, speech production abilities are usually probed through syllable elicitation techniques such as the Phonetic Level Speech Evaluation (Ling 1976) or, for those with sufficiently large expressive vocabularies, through commercially available articulation/phonological tests. An oral mechanism exam is performed to rule out any structural or functional concerns that might interfere with speech development. It is particularly important to assess the child's ability to imitate the Ling (1989) sounds (/m/, /a/, /u/, /i/, /ʃ/ and /s/) before and during the hearing aid trial period. Improved ability to imitate these sounds can be an early indication of benefit from hearing aids.

In summary, the communication assessment provides an estimate of the child's current speech and language abilities relative to those of normally developing children. It can also provide information about the signing proficiency of the child and family members if a signing system is used at home. These pieces of information can give parents and team members a clearer understanding of the child's functional communication abilities. They also provide a baseline for measuring progress during the hearing aid trial and after CI activation.

Psychological Assessments and Counseling

Clinical psychologists participate in the implant decision-making process by completing evaluations of the child's developmental, cognitive, and socio-emotional status. For children under three years, assessments are commonly undertaken through observation, parent reports, and developmental scales such as the *Battelle Developmental Inventory* (2nd Ed., Newborg et al. 2004) or the *Infant-Toddler*

Development Assessment (Provence et al. 1995). Gross and fine motor skills, adaptive behaviors, and nonverbal intelligence are examined to see whether areas not affected by hearing loss or language delays are developing at an expected rate. The child's compliance, cooperation, and social-emotional maturity are also considered.

Psychologists are also instrumental in determining whether children with multiple disabilities can be good candidates for implants. The presence of multiple disabilities (e.g., hearing loss and learning, behavioral, or motoric disabilities) does not necessarily preclude consideration for implantation. For some children with multiple disabilities, receiving an implant may lead to communicative, social, and academic gains beyond what can be expected with hearing aids. Children for whom the implant signal is likely to be perceived as adverse or overly confusing may not be suitable candidates.

The potential advantages and disadvantages of implantation must be identified and weighed carefully before a decision can be made. Psychologists play a key role in this "weighting" process by determining the child's developmental levels and by helping parents and older children consider the range of reasonable outcomes associated with cochlear implant use. Taken together, this information provides parents and team members with a clearer picture of the child's and the family's potential for successful implant use.

Educational Assessments

Educators of children with hearing impairments can provide key information about communication modalities and school-related abilities during the decision-making process. They may help parents select a communication modality (e.g., manually coded English, Cued Speech, or ASL) if one has not been previously chosen. Parental selection of a communication modality requires a clear understanding of the requirements for learning and using each communication modality effectively, and an awareness of available resources—information that educators of children with hearing impairments are specially trained to provide. The family's communication proficiency is also examined whenever a communication system has already been chosen. For children of preschool age and older, school readiness, math, and reading abilities may be assessed. This information is especially useful for selecting initial classroom placements and making educational programming decisions.

Other Issues

The pre-implantation evaluation process varies from center to center. Some centers require many of the tests and procedures described above. Other centers may use only a few selected assessment tools. Some implant programs may require that school placements and intervention services be arranged before setting a surgery date, while others have no firm policy on this issue. Parents who are considering cochlear implantation should contact several implant centers to find out more about testing procedures and follow-up habilitation criteria.

Finally, monetary factors must be considered when making the implant decision. The total cost of receiving a cochlear implant was recently estimated at $55,000 (University of California—San Francisco, Douglas Grant Cochlear Implant Center, 2001) although actual costs vary across the country. This amount includes the pre-operative evaluation, surgery, a short hospital stay, the device itself, and the first year of postoperative treatment (i.e., activation, mapping, and audiological testing). Cochlear implantation is covered by Medicaid and many insurance companies. However, because some insurers do not reimburse for these costs, it is best to verify insurance coverage early in the decision-making process. Further information on insurance reimbursement can be found at *http://www.shhh.org*.

References

Davis, H. and Silverman, S. (1978). *Hearing and deafness* (4th ed.). New York: Holt, Rinehart, & Winston.

Dunn, L. M., Dunn, L. M., and Dunn, D. M. (1997). *Peabody picture vocabulary test* (3rd ed.). Circle Pines, MN: American Guidance Service.

Erber, N. (1982). *Auditory training*. Washington, D.C.: A.G. Bell Association for the Deaf.

Ertmer, D. J. and Mellon, J. A. (2001). Beginning to talk at 20 months: Early vocal development in a young cochlear implant recipient. *Journal of Speech-Language and Hearing Research*, 44, 192-206.

Fenson, L., Dale, P., Resnick, J., and Bates, E. (1993). *MacArthur communication development inventories: User's guide and manual*. San Diego: Singular.

Haskins, H. A. (1949). *A phonetically balanced test of speech discrimination for children*. Northwestern University, Evanston, IL.

Jerger, J., Lewis, S., Hawkins, J., and Jerger, S. (1980). Pediatric speech intelligibility test I: Generation of test materials. *International Journal of Pediatric Otorhynolaryngology*, 2, 101-118.

Kirk, K. I. (2000). Challenges in the clinical investigation of cochlear implant outcomes. In J. Niparko, K. I. Kirk, N. Mellon, A. Robbins, D. Tucci, and B. Wilson (Eds.), *Cochlear implants: Principles and practice* (pp. 225-259). Philadelphia: Lippincott Williams & Wilkins, Inc.

Kirk, K. I., Miyamoto, R. T., Ying, E., Perdew, A. E., and Zuganelis, H. (2002). Cochlear implantation in young children: Effects of age at implantation and communication mode. *Volta Review*, 102, 127-144.

Kirk, K. I., Pisoni, D. B., and Osberger, M. J. (1995). Lexical effects on spoken word recognition in pediatric cochlear implant users. *Ear & Hearing*, 16, 470-481.

Ling, D. (1976). *Speech and the hearing-impaired child: Theory and practice*. Washington, D.C.: A.G. Bell Association.

Ling, D. (1989). *Foundations of spoken language for hearing-impaired children*. Washington, D.C.: A.G. Bell Association.

References, *continued*

Lynch, M. P., Oller, D. K., and Seffans, M. (1989). Development of speech-like vocalizations in a child with congenital absence of cochleas: The case of total deafness. *Applied Psycholinguistics*, 10, 315-333.

Moog, J., Kozak, V., and Geers, A. (1983). *Grammatical analysis of elicited language.* St. Louis, MO: Central Institute for the Deaf.

Moog, J. S. and Geers, A. E. (1990). *Early speech perception test for profoundly hearing-impaired children.* St. Louis: Central Institute for the Deaf.

Nathani, S., Ertmer, D. J., and Stark, R. E. (2002). The stark assessment of early vocal development-revised. Paper presented at the annual convention of the American Speech-Language-Hearing Association, Atlanta, GA.

Newborg, J., Stock, J. R., and Wnek, L. (2004). *Battelle developmental inventory* (2nd ed.). Itasca, IL: Riverside Publishing.

Provence, S., Erikson, J., Vater, S., and Palermi, S. (1995). *Infant – toddler development assessment.* Itasca, IL: Riverside Publishing.

Robbins, A., Renshaw, J. J., Miyamoto, R. T., and Osberger, M. J. (1988). *Minimal pairs test.* Indianapolis, IN: Indiana School of Medicine.

Tucci, D. and Niparko, J. (2000). Medical and surgical aspects of cochlear implantation. In J. Niparko, K. Kirk, J. A. Mellon, A. Robbins, D. Tucci, and B. Wilson (Eds.), *Cochlear implantation: Principles and practices* (pp. 189-224). Philadelphia: Lippincott Williams & Wilkins, Inc.

Tyler, R., Fryhauf-Bertschy, H., and Kelsay, D. (1991). *Children's vowel perception test.* Iowa City: University of Iowa.

Tyler, R. S. (1993). *Cochlear implants: Audiological foundations.* San Diego: Singular.

Waltzman, S. B. and Cohen, N. (1998). Cochlear implantation in children younger than two years old. *American Journal of Otology*, 19, 158-162.

Cochlear Implant Surgery and Activation

3

Once the decision to provide a cochlear implant has been made, a date is set for the surgery. The length of time between the decision and the operation will be determined by the surgeon's schedule and the amount of preparatory work to be completed (e.g., blood tests, audiometric testing, insurance approval). The following is a simplified description of the main steps in the two- to three-hour surgical procedure. Different techniques are used at various implant centers and anatomical abnormalities often require specialized procedures.

The first steps in the implantation process involve anesthetizing the patient, shaving and sterilizing the skin behind the selected ear, and making an incision within the hairline. Next, the skin is laid back and a depression in the mastoid bone is hollowed out to match the size of the internal receiver-stimulator unit. A passageway is then drilled through the bone into the middle ear space. Care must be taken not to damage the facial nerve in the process.

Once the middle ear is accessed, the electrode array is inserted into the cochlea through the round window or through the cochlear wall (i.e., cochleostomy). The array is then guided gently along the basilar membrane in the scala tympany until it is inserted as far as possible within the cochlea. A full insertion is approximately 25–30 mm. For young children, a loop of the electrode cable is coiled near the receiver-stimulator. This "extra" length of cable permits the position of the electrode array in the cochlea to remain undisturbed as the child's head grows. The implant is activated and tested during surgery through inner-operative monitoring. If the internal components work properly, the receiver-stimulator unit and the lead wires are fixed in place with biocompatible cement or sutures, and the incision is closed. X-rays or CT scans may also be taken during surgery to document the position of the internal components.

Children usually spend one night in the hospital and go home the next day if there are no complications. Post-surgical symptoms include pain and stiffness in the neck, a change in taste, and numbness around the incision following surgery. The first two side effects often clear up within a few months, but numbness may persist for a longer time. The implant is usually activated two to six weeks after surgery, giving the child time to recover from the surgical procedure.

Activating the Implant

Activating a cochlear implant is a complex process in which the audiologist introduces a series of very rapid electrical pulses to the auditory nerve through a computer interface with the child's CI. These signals result in a new sensation for the child and may elicit reactions ranging from puzzlement, to fear and crying, to calm acknowledgment. The main goal of this process is to set the voltage levels of the electrodes so that the sensations produced by sound are detectable but not uncomfortable. The amount of electrical current needed to produce a hearing sensation differs from child to child and across the nerve fibers that each electrode stimulates, making each child's first map highly individualized. Implant activation procedures also vary according to the type of implant used. The following is a basic description of the activation process. Interested readers can find more information in Moore and Teagle (2002), Tyler (1993), and in Rance and Dowell (1997).

The first step in the activation process involves fitting the external components of the implant. The speech processor may be worn in a number of locations: on the body in a harness or waist-pack, clipped to the child's clothing, or at ear level. Radio frequency transmitters are held in place over the internal receiver by magnets. The magnetic force needed to hold transmitters in place is adjusted to a comfortable but secure level.

Figure 3.1: Child with body CI	Figure 3.2: Child with MED-EL clip-on processor	Figure 3.3: Child with ear-level processor
	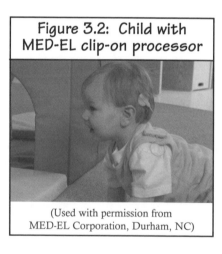	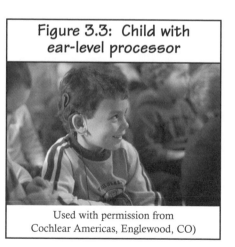
	(Used with permission from MED-EL Corporation, Durham, NC)	Used with permission from Cochlear Americas, Englewood, CO)

(Used with permission from Advanced Bionics, Inc., Sylmar, CA)

The activation process often requires two professionals: an audiologist who uses computer software to present the signal and another person (generally an audiologist or SLP) to hold the child's attention and watch for the responses when electrodes are activated. Parents and observers are cautioned not to distract the child or indicate when the stimulating pulses are presented.

Several tasks are completed during the initial activation process. First, the audiologist selects a stimulating mode for the implant by setting the desired distance between the active and the ground electrodes. In effect, stimulation modes determine the size of the area over which receptor nerve cells are stimulated and influence the amount of electrical current needed to produce a hearing response. Stimulating modes differ according to implant models. Table 3.1 lists the main kinds of modes available.

Table 3.1: Stimulating Modes for Multi-channel Cochlear Implants	
Stimulating Mode	Description
Common Ground	Electrical current flows from active electrodes to a ball-shaped electrode placed in the temporalis muscle or to non-active electrodes within the array.
Monopolar	Electrical current flows from active electrodes to a single electrode that remains outside of the cochlea, creating a wide distribution of energy.
Bipolar	The active and the ground electrode are next to each other, creating a narrow distribution of energy.
Bipolar +1	The active and the ground electrode are separated by an intermediary electrode, a commonly used mode with a relatively narrow focus.
Bipolar +2	The active and the ground electrode are separated by two intermediary electrodes, creating a wider distribution of energy than bipolar or bipolar +1.

A second task involves setting the voltage levels for each electrode. This process is commonly called "mapping" or "programming" the implant. CI maps control the minimum and maximum amounts of voltage that individual electrodes deliver to the auditory nerve. These amounts are determined by measuring the electrical threshold and comfort levels exhibited by the child. Electrical thresholds are identified by gradually increasing the amount of voltage emitted by an electrode until the child produces a consistent, observable response. This is accomplished by using procedures similar to those for measuring unaided and aided hearing levels prior to implantation (i.e., visual reinforcement audiometry and conditioned play audiometry).

Comfort levels are equivalent to the maximum amount of stimulation that can be presented without discomfort. For young children, initial comfort levels are usually set slightly above threshold levels to avoid discomfort and permit gradual acclimatization to sound. Once threshold and comfort levels have been established for a few electrodes, computer programs can be used to set the output levels for the remaining channels. The initial map produces a signal that is unlikely to be rejected by the child.

The child's dynamic range (the difference in voltage between threshold and comfort levels) is a key measure of CI benefit. Although dynamic range is usually small in the child's first map, later mapping sessions seek to lower thresholds and increase acceptance of higher voltage levels, helping the child to detect softer sounds and tolerate louder ones. Compared to children with normal hearing, those with cochlear implants typically have a much smaller dynamic range (120 dB SPL vs. approximately 24 dB SPL respectively, Moore and Teagle 2002). Because better speech perception abilities have been associated with wider dynamic ranges in children with CIs (Geers 2002), a major goal of mapping sessions is to increase the child's dynamic range.

Once mapping has been completed, the outputs of the electrodes are balanced so that voltage ranges are similar across the array. For older children and adults, this usually involves asking the CI user to judge the loudness of the signal produced by individual or groups of electrodes (i.e., loudness scaling). A similar process may be used to assess the perception of pitch associated with electrodes from the basal (those with high frequency representation) to apical locations (those with low frequency representation) along the basilar membrane. This procedure is called *pitch ranking* and requires the CI user to judge whether signals are higher or lower in pitch as electrodes are activated. Computer programs are used to balance electrode output for young children who are not cognitively or linguistically mature enough to participate in these activities.

After the computer-controlled stimuli have been presented, it's time for the child to respond to actual sounds and speech. This is the moment that parents have been waiting for. Some children, however, become distressed by the unfamiliar sensations and react with tears and confusion. It is important that parents be aware of this possibility prior to activation, so that their interactions with the child can be calm and encouraging. During this first listening experience, parent and clinician voices should be of moderate intensity as they speak with the child, calling his or her name, or saying short sentences. Environmental sounds and toys that make pleasant sounds can also be introduced. These experiences should be monitored closely so that the child's first exposure to sound is positive and not overwhelming.

As the activation session comes to a close, parents are given a suggested schedule for use of the CI. This usually entails wearing the device for one to two hours in quiet environments at first. Care should be taken to avoid loud noises and noisy environments that seem to upset the child. The duration and the variety of listening situations can be gradually increased over the next month until the child is wearing the CI during all waking hours.

Parents typically have many questions at this stage of the session. Table 3.2 on page 40 contains a list of important items for discussion (Mecklenberg et al. 1990). The answers to these questions, as well as maintenance and warranty information, can be found in the owner's manual of the child's device. The activation session ends as parents are provided with the audiologist's phone number and instructed to contact the implant center if they have additional questions or concerns.

Table 3.2: Common Questions About Cochlear Implants

▶ How is the speech processor turned on and off?

▶ How are batteries changed?

▶ How long should batteries last?

▶ Can rechargeable batteries be used?

▶ How is the speech processor tested to see if it's working properly?

▶ What does the sensitivity control do?

▶ Can the speech processor be repaired?

▶ How can the speech processor be connected to a FM or infrared assistive listening system?

▶ How can the telephone signal be fed into the speech processor?

▶ How can the television sound be fed into the speech processor?

(Adapted from Mecklenberg et al. 1990)

Routine Mapping

Children typically return for a second mapping session approximately one month after CI activation. This session has the following purposes:

▶ to assess the child's acceptance of the CI

▶ to determine whether technical problems have been experienced

▶ to answer parent questions

▶ to support parents in the use of the CI and in the development of listening skills

▶ to determine threshold and comfort levels for electrodes not tested during previous sessions

▶ to increase dynamic range by providing new maps, as tolerated by the child

▶ to observe the child's reactions to speech and environmental sounds

▶ to determine CI hearing thresholds and speech detection levels

▶ to begin speech perception testing, if possible.

Although implant centers vary in the frequency of appointments, follow-up mapping sessions are usually scheduled at three-, six-, and twelve-month intervals during the first year of implant use and at six-month or one-year intervals thereafter. These sessions have the same general purposes as the first post-activation session. In addition, parents are instructed to contact the implant center for an appointment if their child encounters any technical or implant-related health problems between appointments.

Children should show gradual improvements in listening, speaking, and oral language use as cochlear implant experience is gained and dynamic range is expanded. The rate at which these improvements are made can be influenced by factors such as age at implantation, aided hearing levels, length of deafness, age at onset of deafness, cognitive abilities, reliability of the CI, and quality of intervention services. Parents, clinicians, and members of the implant team must work together to monitor progress so that any necessary adjustments to the implant or to the child's intervention program can be made as soon as possible.

Being a Part of the CI Team

School-based professionals and early interventionists can be useful adjunct members of the CI team. Because they see the child on a regular basis, they are often the first to notice progress and identify concerns. Moore and Teagle (2002) point out several important ways that communication interventionists can, with the permission of the parents, be active members of the CI team. Their suggestions include:

▶ attending pre- and post-implantation appointments with the family

▶ sharing information about the child's communication status, hearing history, and educational placement

▶ supporting parents in developing realistic expectations for the amount of time and effort needed to help their child learn to use hearing for communication

▶ ensuring consistent use of the CI at school and at home

Conversely, professionals from the implant center can promote the aural habilitation process by sharing the results of mapping and testing sessions, providing advice on technology issues (e.g., fitting Assistive Listening Devices, or trouble-shooting), and responding to the questions of the interventionist. Collaboration between the family and all involved professionals is essential for making well-informed decisions regarding communication modalities and educational placements—the topics of Chapter 4.

References

Geers, A. E. (2002). Factors affecting the development of speech, language, and literacy in children with early cochlear implantation. *Language, Speech, and Hearing Services in Schools*, 33, 172-183.

Mecklenburg, D., Blamey, P., Busby, P., Dowell, R., Roberts, S., and Rickarts, F. (1990). Auditory (re)habilitation for implanted deaf children and teenagers. In G. Clark, Y. Tong, and J. Patrick (Eds.), *Cochlear prostheses* (pp. 207-222). New York: Churchill Livingston.

Moore, J. A. and Teagle, H. F. B. (2002). An introduction to cochlear implant technology, activation, and programming. *Language, Speech, and Hearing Services in Schools*, 33, 153-161.

Rance, G. and Dowell, R. C. (1997). Speech processor programming. In G. M. Clark, R. S. C. Cowan, and R. C. Dowell (Eds.), *Cochlear implantation for infants and children: Advances* (pp. 147-170). San Diego: Singular.

Tyler, R. S. (1993). *Cochlear implants: Audiological foundations*. San Diego: Singular.

Communication Modalities and Educational Placements for Children with CIs

4

To Sign or Not to Sign?

The merits of various methods for communicating with children who are deaf have been passionately debated for hundreds of years. Although strong preferences continue to be championed today, professionals are finding that a family-centered approach to choosing a communication modality can help parents understand their options, empower them to make appropriate choices for their families, and encourage them to become advocates for their children (Moeller and Condon 1998).

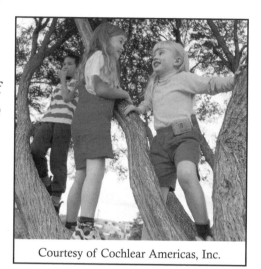

Courtesy of Cochlear Americas, Inc.

In a family-centered approach, parents and professionals view themselves as partners in a problem-solving process. To achieve this level of collaboration, professionals strive to form genuine relationships with parents so that their feelings and concerns can be discussed openly. They also provide objective information about a full range of communication modalities. Parents are encouraged to choose the communication option that is best-suited for their child and their family after they have acquired an understanding of the pros and cons of each approach.

Two definitions are helpful for understanding the relationship between children's hearing levels and their communication options. For the purposes of this discussion, the term *deaf* is used to describe the hearing status of children with profound hearing loss in both ears (i.e., three frequency pure-tone thresholds greater than 90 dB HL). Children with hearing losses of this magnitude typically have very limited access to speech at conversational intensity levels—even with hearing aids. The term *hard of hearing* is used to describe the status of children with mild-to-severe hearing losses in one or both ears (i.e., three frequency pure-tone thresholds ranging between 21–90 dB HL). Children with residual hearing in this range have relatively greater potential to become oral communicators via hearing aids because they have better access to conversational speech.

The ages at which children become deaf can also influence the selection of a communication modality. Children who are born deaf are said to have *congenital* hearing losses. They have never had auditory access to speech. Children who become deaf between birth and two years of age are said to have *prelingual* deafness because their hearing loss began before or during the very early stages of language development. These children have had little or no exposure to the sounds of speech before the onset of deafness. In contrast, children who lose their hearing later in life can often use their previous listening and speaking experiences to maintain and expand their oral communication abilities. The remainder of this chapter will focus on communication modalities and educational placement options for children who are prelingually deaf and use cochlear implants.

Three communication modalities are commonly used in the United States: Oral Communication, Total Communication, and bilingual use of American Sign Language and English. The main features of these communication options and their advantages and disadvantages for children with CIs will be highlighted below. Cued Speech, a manual system to supplement speechreading, will also be considered. Finally, this chapter presents an overview of educational placements for children with hearing loss and a list of suggested readings and Internet resources.

Oral Communication

Contemporary supporters of Oral Communication (OC) believe that children who are deaf can learn to listen and talk by using hearing aids or cochlear implants and receiving auditory, speech production, spoken language, and speechreading training. This philosophy is also known as an Auditory-Oral or Oral approach (Ling 1964). A second group of OC supporters, those that endorse the Auditory-Verbal method, agrees with this basic premise but opts to remove tactile and speechreading cues from intervention activities. This unisensory approach is based on the belief that focusing solely on auditory information will result in more efficient development of listening and oral communication skills (Bebee et al. 1984). The availability of educational programs with an OC philosophy has increased as the age criteria for cochlear implantation has decreased. According to the Oral Deaf Education Web site (Oraldeaf.com), there are approximately 40 private oral schools in the U.S. Public school systems are also adding OC programs for children with hearing loss, and correspondence courses in English and Spanish are available through the John Tracy Clinic (see Web site address at the end of this chapter). The characteristics of Auditory-Oral and Auditory-Verbal programs can be found in Table 4.1 on pages 46 and 47.

Table 4.1: Communication Modalities Described

	American Sign Language/English as a Second Language (ASL/ESL) Bilingual/Bicultural	Auditory-Verbal Unisensory	Cued Speech	Oral Auditory-Oral	Total Communication
Definition	A manual language that is distinct from spoken English (ASL is not based on English grammar/syntax). Extensively used within and among the deaf community. English is taught as a second language.	A program emphasizing auditory skills. Teaches a child to develop listening skills through one-on-one therapy that focuses attention on use of remaining hearing (with the aid of amplification). Since this method strives to make the most of a child's listening abilities, no manual communication is used and the child is discouraged from relying on visual cues.	A visual communication system of eight hand shapes (cues) that represent different sounds of speech. These cues are used while talking to make the spoken language clear through vision. This system allows the child to distinguish sounds that look the same on the lips.	Program that teaches a child to make maximum use of his/her remaining hearing through amplification (hearing aids, cochlear implant, FM system). This program also stresses the use of speech reading to aid the child's communication. Use of any form of manual communication (sign language) is not encouraged although natural gestures may be supported.	Philosophy of using every and all means to communicate with deaf children. The child is exposed to a formal sign-language system (based on English), finger spelling (manual alphabet), natural gestures, speech reading, body language, oral speech and use of amplification. The idea is to communicate and teach vocabulary and language in any manner that works.
Primary Goals	To be the deaf child's primary language and allow him/her to communicate before learning to speak or even if the child never learns to speak effectively. Since ASL is commonly referred to as "the language of the deaf," it prepares the child for social access to the deaf community.	To develop speech, primarily through the use of aided hearing alone, and communication skills necessary for integration into the hearing community.	To develop speech and communication skills necessary for integration into the hearing community.	To develop speech and communication skills necessary for integration into the hearing community.	To provide an easy, least restrictive communication method between the deaf child and his/her family, teachers and schoolmates. The child's simultaneous use of speech and sign language is encouraged as is use of all other visual and contextual cues.
Language Development (Receptive)	Language is developed through the use of ASL. English is taught as a second language after the child has mastered ASL.	Child learns to speak through the early, consistent and successful use of a personal amplification system (hearing aids, cochlear implant, FM system).	Child learns to speak through the use of amplification, speech reading and use of "cues" which represent different sounds.	Child learns to speak through a combination of early, consistent and successful use of amplification and speech reading.	Language (be it spoken or sign or a combination of the two) is developed through exposure to oral speech, a formal sign language system, speech reading and the use of an amplification system.
Expressive Language	ASL is child's primary expressive language in addition to written English.	Spoken and written English.	Spoken English (sometimes with the use of cues) and written English.	Spoken and written English.	Spoken English and/or sign language and finger spelling and written English

Table 4.1: Communication Modalities Described, *continued*

	American Sign Language/ English as a Second Language (ASL/ESL) *Bilingual/Bicultural*	Auditory-Verbal *Unisensory*	Cued Speech	Oral *Auditory-Oral*	Total Communication
Hearing	Use of amplification is not a requirement for success with ASL.	Early, consistent and successful use of amplification (hearing aids, cochlear implant, FM system) is critical to this approach.	Use of amplification is strongly encouraged to maximize the use of remaining hearing.	Early and consistent use of amplification (hearing aids, cochlear implant, FM system) is critical to this method.	Use of a personal amplification system (hearing aids, cochlear implant, FM system) is strongly encouraged to allow child to make the most of his/her remaining hearing.
Family Responsibility	Child must have access to deaf and/or hearing adults who are fluent in ASL in order to develop this as a primary language. If the parents choose this method they will need to communicate with their child fully.	Since the family is primarily responsible for the child's language development, parents are expected to incorporate on-going training into the child's daily routine and play activities. They must provide a language-rich environment, make hearing a meaningful part of all the child's experiences and ensure full-time use of amplification.	Parents are the primary teachers of cued speech to their child. They are expected to cue at all times while they speak; consequently, at least one parent, and preferably both, must learn to cue fluently for the child to develop age-appropriate speech & language.	Since the family is primarily responsible for the child's language development, parents are expected to incorporate training and practice sessions (learned from therapists) into the child's daily routine and play activities. In addition, the family is responsible for ensuring consistent use of amplification.	At least one, but preferably all family members, should learn the chosen sign language system in order for the child to develop age-appropriate language and communicate fully with his/her family. It should be noted that a parent's acquisition of sign vocabulary and language is a long term, ongoing process. As the child's expressive sign language broadens and becomes more complex, so too should the parents' in order to provide the child with a stimulating language learning environment. The family is also responsible for encouraging consistent use of amplification.
Parent Training	If parents are not deaf, intensive ASL training and education about deaf culture is desired in order for the family to become proficient in the language.	Parents need to be highly involved with child's teacher and/or therapists (speech, auditory-verbal, etc.) in order to learn training methods and carry them over to the home environment.	Cued speech can be learned through classes taught by trained teachers or therapists. A significant amount of time must be spent using and practicing cues to become proficient.	Parents need to be highly involved with child's teacher and/or therapists (speech, aural habilitation, etc.) to carry over training activities to the home and create an optimal "oral" learning environment. These training activities would emphasize development of listening, speech reading and speech skills.	Parents must consistently sign when they speak to their child (simultaneous communication). Sign language courses are routinely offered through the community, local colleges, adult education, etc. Additionally, many books and videos are widely available. To become fluent, signing must be used consistently and become a routine part of your communication.

Courtesy of Beginnings for Parents of Children Who Are Deaf or Hard of Hearing (www.beginningssvcs.com)

The primary goals of cochlear implantation are to improve hearing sensitivity and speech perception ability. Secondary benefits in speech production and oral language development can be expected as auditory abilities increase. Although there is considerable variability in the amount of progress made, research has shown that the combination of consistent CI use and clinical intervention leads to significant improvements in listening, speaking, and language skills for most children (see Kirk 2002 for review). Advocates of OC believe that progress can be optimized when spoken language is the sole form of communication at home, in therapy, and in school.

Adopting an OC approach also simplifies communication for most families. Because 90% of children who are deaf are born to hearing parents, choosing OC enables families to stimulate language development without having to learn an additional form of communication. Similarly, children who become proficient oral communicators have a shared channel of communication with peers who have normal hearing. On the other hand, adults who take signing classes often find them enriching and enjoy signing with their children.

Although OC is well-aligned with the objectives of cochlear implantation and the communication capabilities of most families, concerns and limitations must also be acknowledged. To begin with, choosing OC means that parent-child communication is limited to gestures, eye-gaze, and physical contact prior to the time the implant is activated. Young children whose parents use manual signs and speech have been shown to have larger vocabularies than those who rely on OC (Schafer and Lynch 1980). To address this concern, some parents may choose to use manual signs with their children before and during the initial months of implant use.

Parents should also have a realistic understanding of the factors that affect auditory learning with a CI. First, it is important to remember that children who receive CIs do not hear normally. In most cases, they have aided hearing levels that are poorer-than-normal in the implanted ear and little or no usable hearing in the other ear. Although their implant hearing levels are better than could be expected with HAs, use of a CI requires ongoing refinement of the implant map, concerted efforts to provide quiet listening environments for learning, and the use of assistive listening devices (e.g., FM or infrared listening systems) to overcome noise and reverberation in group settings.

In contrast to typically developing children who acquire spoken language without direct instruction, prelingually deaf children with CIs require extensive instruction and practice to develop oral communication skills. Geers (2002) found that the 136 school-age children she studied averaged 80–90 minutes of communication intervention per week during their first four years of implant use. Toddlers and preschoolers are also likely to need intensive intervention if they are to maximize learning during a sensitive period for language acquisition (Ryugo et al. 2000). These needs can be met as parents employ language stimulation strategies throughout the day and clinicians offer support and direct intervention as the child matures.

Finally, it must be remembered that some children experience considerable auditory learning difficulties despite improved hearing sensitivity and intensive intervention. These children may learn to communicate more readily when spoken language is augmented with a signing system. The combination of spoken language and manual signs will be explored next.

Total Communication

In its original form, Total Communication (TC) was designed to encourage communicators to use a variety of means to exchange ideas with deaf children (Scouten 1984). Parents and teachers who used this approach were instructed to speak, gesture, sign, write, fingerspell, draw pictures, or use a combination of these means to communicate with deaf children.

In its current application, TC usually refers to the production of speech and signs together, and can more accurately be described as Simultaneous Communication or "Sim-Com." This form of TC requires the message sender to match spoken words and grammatical markers (e.g., word prefixes and suffixes) with manually-signed and finger-spelled counterparts. The main premise of this approach is that the combination of auditory and visual information will enable children to learn spoken English more efficiently than using either form of communication alone (see Table 4.1 on pages 46 and 47). In the U.S., TC requires the use of some form of manually-coded English (e.g., Signed English or Signing Exact English), enabling parents and siblings to use their native language to communicate with their children. When applied to children with CIs and hearing aids, TC is intended to facilitate listening, speech, and oral language development while providing a visually accessible representation of vocabulary and language constructions. Today, approximately 66% of the educational programs available for children with hearing loss use a TC approach (Schow and Nerbonne 2002).

Although TC is intended to provide a user-friendly method of communicating, in practice, the correspondence between what is spoken and what is signed can be difficult to coordinate. This difficulty begins to come into play as ideas are expressed in sentences. Up until that point, the production of single signs and two-word sign combinations with speech is relatively straightforward. However, as ideas become more complex and grammatical markers are used (e.g., for verb tense, possession, and plurality), the string of words, signs, and finger-spelled markers becomes longer and more difficult to produce and understand. In addition, TC users may slow or distort their speech because of limited signing skills, providing unnatural models of speech. These difficulties can cause TC users to simplify and shorten messages, giving children a telegraphic model rather than a well-formed example of an English sentence (Luetke-Stahlman 1991). In addition to concerns about coordinating speech and sign, TC parents must continually learn many new signs and grammatical structures if they are to stay a "step ahead" of their children.

Despite these potential difficulties, many families use TC to communicate successfully, and many deaf children with CIs develop functional speech and sign skills. It is also important to remember that there are options in adopting a TC approach. Some parents begin to use TC with their children before CI activation and continue thereafter. Others gradually decrease signing as the child becomes more reliant on hearing and oral language skills. As Robbins (2000) notes, children with implants who use TC may become quite adept at oral communication in predictable situations at home and with peers. They may, however, continue to rely on signing interpreters to succeed in their schoolwork. The suggestions in Table 4.2 are offered for parents who wish to begin using TC with their children.

Table 4.2: Suggestions for Normally Hearing Parents with Young Children Who Use Manual Signs

▶ Begin with a few key signs and phrases that allow you to communicate with your child.

▶ Be sure you have your child's attention as you begin to sign.

▶ Practice understanding a variety of signers, including both adults and children.

▶ Expand your signing skills to include more complex utterances and new vocabulary.

▶ Strive to sign at a higher level than your child in terms of vocabulary diversity and the number of signs combined.

▶ Develop fluency by signing at a steady rate and avoiding "breaks" in the message.

▶ Use inflection in your signing, especially when reading or telling stories.

▶ Encourage all family members to sign with your child.

(Adapted from Moeller et al. 1994)

Research on OC and TC in Children with Cochlear Implants

Over the last decade, researchers have begun to examine the influence of OC and TC on the development of speech perception, speech production, and language skills after cochlear implantation. The following is a synthesis of key findings in these areas for children with prelingual deafness.

Recent research shows that implanted children who use OC make greater and more rapid progress in developing speech perception abilities than those who use TC (Geers 2002, Kirk et al. 2002, Osberger and Fischer 2000, and Tobey et al. 2000). The uniformity of these research outcomes indicates that an oral approach is superior to the use of speech and sign for the development of auditory perceptual skills. The clear advantage of OC also suggests that children who use TC may need extra emphasis to reach their speech perception potentials. Barker et al. (1997, p. 174) recommend that "at least some time each day" be spent focusing on the auditory signal (without supplemental signs) to optimize their speech perception abilities.

Although somewhat mixed, investigations of speech development also support OC as advantageous over TC. Osberger et al. (1994) reported considerably better speech intelligibility for OC children than TC children (mean scores of 48% vs. 21% words understood, respectively). The children in this study were fit with their devices at a mean age of 4:0 and 4:4, respectively, and had at least two years of CI experience. Tobey et al. (2000) reported a comparable advantage in intelligibility for OC vs. TC children who had used their devices for four to six years (mean scores of 50% vs. 30% respectively). In contrast to the advantage noted for OC, Conner et al. (2000) found that OC and TC users produced consonants with comparable accuracy. Speech development is a complex process that can be examined at many levels. The first two studies indicate that children who use OC make more rapid progress in developing functional speech skills than children who use TC. The latter investigation suggests that the two groups may acquire some basic speech skills at an equivalent rate.

No clear advantage for either OC or TC has been observed when several recent studies of language development are considered. In each of these investigations, language tests were administered in the child's mode of communication. Geers (2002, p. 180) found comparable "Total Language" scores (derived from a battery of measures) among OC and TC users who were implanted by five years of age and had four to six years of CI experience. Comparable rates of development in receptive language abilities were also documented for the two groups by Kirk et al. (2002). The latter investigation used the *Reynell Developmental Language Scales* (*RDLS*) with children implanted before five years. In contrast, two recent studies have detected a relative advantage for one or the other modality. Conner et al. (2000) found that TC children with six months to ten years of CI experience had greater vocabulary growth than OC children with similar lengths of CI use. The Kirk et al. (2002) study determined that OC children made more rapid gains in expressive language abilities than TC children on the RDLS. Further research is needed to determine whether either communication modality has a consistent advantage for spoken language development.

Cued Speech

Cued Speech was developed at Gallaudet University by Cornet (1967) as a manual supplement for speechreading (see Table 4.1 on pages 46 and 47). The intent of Cued Speech (CS) is to reduce the speechreading confusion caused by speech sounds that look the same on the lips (e.g., /p/, /b/, /m/) and those that lack visual cues altogether (e.g., /t/, /d/, /k/, /g/). In this system, a hand is placed in one of four positions near the chin and the mouth. These hand positions represent sets of English vowels. Eight hand shapes are formed through combinations of raised fingers to represent sets of consonants.

Each speech sound within a particular vowel or consonant set is visually distinct from all others within the set (i.e., has a different lip or mouth shape). For example, placing the hand near the chin represents either /o/, /e/, or /u/ (vowels that differ in lip rounding). A hand shape with all five fingers extended represents either /t/, /m/, or /f/ (consonants with visibly distinguishable places of articulation). Hand shape and placement cues are presented in combination as their corresponding speech sounds are spoken.

Several characteristics of Cued Speech support its adoption for children who have CIs. First, CS facilitates communication by allowing "cuers" to make use of their residual hearing, speechreading ability, and knowledge of manual cues to understand messages. Conversely, speech and manual cues are used for self-expression. Thus, CS takes advantage of the child's improved auditory capabilities and encourages intelligible speech. Secondly, parents may find learning to "cue" is easier than learning a sign system/language because a small number of manual cues represent all English phonemes. Rather than having to learn signs for thousands of words or the grammar of a visual-gestural language, cuers can convey the phonemic characteristics of each word using eight hand shapes, four hand placements, and diphthong movements. Finally, by emphasizing the identity of vowels and consonants in words, CS increases phonemic awareness and may contribute to the development of literacy skills.

Vernon and Andrews (1990) have noted some difficulties in using CS as a communication system. Three cited concerns are relevant for children with CIs. First, the receiver must be a good speechreader to interpret cues. Young CI recipients who are prelingually deaf, however, do not have well-developed speechreading skills because they are just beginning to acquire spoken language. It is not known how the simultaneous presentation of three signals (i.e., auditory, speechreading, and manual cues) will impact early language learning. Secondly, group communication can be difficult for "cuers" because manual and speech-reading cues are less accessible from the side of the speaker. Thirdly, cues for homophenous words (i.e., words that look the same on the lips such as *cough* and *golf*) can be difficult to interpret. Additionally, communication is restricted when others do not know the cues. Little is known about the effects of using CS with prelingually deaf toddlers who have cochlear implants. Children who lose their hearing later in life (e.g., after three years) may be better able to learn CS, at least initially, because of their relatively stronger language base.

Parents who choose this approach will need special training and local support to develop and refine their skills. Likewise, children who use CS should interact regularly with other cuers so that they can improve their skills as well. Classroom CS interpreters may be needed throughout the child's school career. Cued Speech programs are not offered in all parts of the country. Information on the availability of services can be found through the National Cued Speech Association.

American Sign Language

Supporters of American Sign Language (ASL) believe that children who are deaf will acquire an auditory-oral language more efficiently when they learn a visual-gestural language first so that one language (ASL) can be used in the bilingual development of the other. ASL is a rule-governed, visual-gestural language (Paul 2001) and is one of the many sign languages used throughout the world. It has both manual (i.e., precise hand configurations, movements, locations, and orientations) and non-manual features (i.e., movements of the head, eyes, lips, and eyebrows). The linguistic structure of ASL is quite different from that of English, making it impossible to communicate with ASL and speak English at the same time. ASL has no written form; users learn to read and write the English language (see Table 4.1, pages 46 and 47).

Recently, a Bilingual-Bicultural (Bi-Bi) model for educating children who are deaf has gained acceptance in the U.S. (Johnson et al. 1990). In this approach, parents begin to learn ASL soon after the child's hearing loss is detected and native ASL users interact with the family so that mature signing models can be presented to the child from a young age. The family is also introduced to deaf culture (persons with hearing loss who share a common set of traditions, values, and history) so that the child can begin to develop an identity within that culture as well as in the hearing world.

A major premise of the Bi-Bi approach is that establishing ASL as a first language will enable children to more easily learn to read and write English as a second language (Paul 2001). Accordingly, ASL is used for everyday communication and classroom instruction. The development of spoken English skills is addressed through classroom curriculum and communication training sessions. ASL users have access to oral communication models through hearing members of their families and their hearing acquaintances. ASL and Bi-Bi programs are found mainly in large cities and at state-run schools for deaf children. More information on ASL, Deaf culture, and educational options can be found through the National Association for the Deaf.

There are several fundamental problems with adopting ASL as a means of communication for children with CIs. The first concern has to do with the lack of auditory information exchanged between ASL users. In ASL, communication among adult signers typically occurs without speech. As a result, an ASL approach does not take advantage of the improved hearing sensitivity that CIs provide. Secondly, learning sign language through an unimpaired visual system is likely to be easier than learning spoken language with improved, though less than optimal, hearing ability. The ease with which ideas can be shared through signing may make CI recipients less attentive to and less reliant on audition for communication. If this is the case, children who interact primarily with ASL users may not be fully engaged in the effortful task of developing auditory, speech, and oral language skills.

Finally, there is an apparent mismatch between the long-range goals of cochlear implantation and the amount of attention paid to oral communication in a Bi-Bi approach. Most hearing parents choose cochlear implantation because they want their children to become participating members of society at large. Reaching this goal requires competence in oral communication. Such competence is not likely to be achieved without abundant oral communication experiences and practice beginning at a young age. By emphasizing sign language early in life and providing comparatively fewer spoken language opportunities, Bi-Bi programs might not provide sufficient support for developing oral communication competence and participation in mainstream society.

Despite these concerns, some parents do decide that the combination of a CI and ASL makes sense for their child and family. For example, they might wish their child to have unimpeded communication through a visual-gestural language and have improved hearing for essential communication and environmental safety reasons. These parents may also believe that involvement in Deaf culture is important for the social and emotional well-being of their child. If so, they may be willing to accept the limited emphasis on auditory, speech, and oral communication found in a Bi-Bi approach.

Professionals who are true to a family-centered approach to counseling and intervention should support such decisions when the parents clearly understand the advantages and disadvantages of their choice and have realistic expectations for their child's communication outcomes. This support includes continued technical assistance, suggestions for maximizing benefit from the implant, and regular exchanges of information with school personnel. Enrollment in a supplemental aural habilitation program can also be arranged for children who wish to develop oral communication skills, as well as ASL. In short, collaboration among implant team members, interventionists, educators, and parents must have the same degree of dedication, regardless of the chosen mode of communication.

Selecting a Communication Modality

In summary, the choice of a communication modality is influenced by many factors, including the child's learning style, parental preferences, and/or the local availability of programs that support each modality. Each of these factors must be carefully considered if parents are to make the best choice for their child and family. Professionals contribute to the decision-making process by providing a supportive relationship, unbiased information, resources that explain communication options, and opportunities to meet families who have adopted each modality. Successful use of a family-centered approach can also lead to greater parent involvement in early intervention programs and increased advocacy throughout the school years.

Educational Placements

Infants and Toddlers

Public law 99-457 (Education of Handicapped Act Amendment 1986) has mandated that early education services (including audiologic, speech-language, and aural habilitation) be provided for children under the age of 5.0 who have significant developmental delays or disabilities. As a result, state and local education agencies are required to identify and supply services for young children at-risk for learning problems. Now that hearing loss can be identified through newborn hearing screening, babies are regularly enrolled in parent-infant programs that provide information, counseling, and guidance in the context of a family-centered approach. The nature of these services will be described in detail in Chapter 6.

Parent-infant programs are available through state and local agencies and professionals in private practice. The former programs are typically provided at reduced cost to families. The cost of private therapy is often, but not always, covered by the family's health insurance policy. It is essential that family-centered intervention begin as soon as possible after a hearing loss is identified. Research has shown that children who receive intervention services by 11 months of age develop better language skills than those who begin to receive services later in life (Moeller 2000).

Preschool Program

It is quite common for children with CIs to begin attending regular preschools or preschools for children with hearing loss at three years of age. Regular preschools follow typical developmental and school-readiness curricula and are taught by early childhood educators. They also provide abundant opportunities for children with CIs to interact with normally hearing peers. Support services for auditory, speech, and language development, and a sign interpreter (if needed) are arranged through the local school district.

Special arrangements and strategies are needed to optimize learning in a regular preschool. Teachers should receive in-service training on how to care for the implant (to be covered in Chapter 5) and given strategies to ensure good communication (e.g., getting the child's attention before talking, enunciating clearly, speaking slightly louder than normal, and communicating face-to-face whenever possible). Preferential seating should also be arranged for each instructional activity. The child's audiologist can help to fit Assistive Listening Devices (ALDs) for use in the classroom and suggest environmental modifications to reduce noise and reverberation (see Chapter 9).

Special preschools for children with hearing loss are well-designed to meet the needs of children with CIs. The advantages of preschools for children with hearing impairments include:

▶ teachers who are specially trained in OC, TC, ASL, or Cued Speech (depending on the school's philosophy)

▶ a curriculum that addresses both pre-academic and communication needs

▶ availability of audiology and speech-language services

▶ acoustically treated classrooms and the availability of ALDs

▶ parent support groups

▶ options for enrollment in "in-house" kindergarten and first grade classrooms to prepare children for regular classroom placement

▶ a liaison teacher to coordinate children's transitions to regular elementary school placements

In many cases, toddlers can transition from family-centered intervention to a preschool classroom within the same local program. An in-depth description of the workings of an oral school can be found in Wilkins and Ertmer (2002). Ideas for helping preschoolers improve their listening, speaking, and language skills will be presented in Chapter 7.

School-Age Children

Table 4.3 provides a range of educational placements for school-age children with hearing loss. The placements are ordered from least to most integrated with regular education programs. A variety of communication modalities can be used in each setting. Children receiving Auditory-Verbal training are usually integrated into regular classrooms.

A recent survey of 35 school-age CI recipients (Niparko et al. 2000) found that most children were enrolled in self-contained classrooms for children with hearing loss prior to implantation and for the first two years of implant use. The authors propose that continued enrollment in special classrooms after implantation is necessary for developing a base of communication and (pre)academic skills. A trend toward increased integration in regular classrooms was observed after the children had three years of implant experience. By the end of year four, approximately 75% of children with CIs were enrolled in mainstream classrooms, the majority for the entire day.

Niparko and colleagues (2000) also noted that the amount of support services needed by children with CIs who were fully mainstreamed was only a quarter of the amount received by a comparison group of deaf children who used hearing aids. Decreased reliance on special education classrooms and support services is, of course, good news for parents because it signals significant academic and social progress. It is also good news for local school districts because greater inclusion in regular education programs leads to significant cost savings over time.

Table 4.3: Educational Placement Options for Children with Hearing Loss	
Residential Schools	State-run or private schools with dormitories for students. Most students live on campus throughout the week and go home on weekends. Some students live at home and commute to classes daily.
Day Schools	A school in which all of the children have hearing loss. Students commute or are bussed to the school each day. Day schools are usually found in large cities.
Day Classes or Self-contained Classrooms	Classes of children with hearing loss are located within a regular school. Children are mainstreamed into regular classrooms for academic content as appropriate.
Partial Mainstreaming	Placement in a regular classroom on a part-time basis. Individualized instruction for some academic areas is provided in a resource room for children with hearing loss or in a resource room for children with a variety of special educational needs.
Inclusion in Regular Classrooms	Enrollment in classrooms with normally hearing peers. Academic, speech and language, and interpreter support are provided as needed for success in the regular classroom.

Optimizing the benefits of cochlear implantation requires much hard work on part of children, parents, and professionals. In addition to the special educational programming described above, several basic procedures are needed to be sure that the cochlear implant works properly everyday. Guidelines for caring for the implant are presented in the upcoming chapter.

Suggested Reading

Choices in Deafness (2nd Edition)
Schwartz, S., Ph.D. (1996)
Woodbine House

Cochlear Implants for Kids
Estabrooks, W. (1998)
A.G. Bell Association

Early Use of Total Communication: An Introductory Guide for Parents
Gibbs, E. D., Springer, A., and Gibbs, B. (1995)
Paul H. Brookes Publishing

Kid Friendly Parenting with Deaf and Hard of Hearing Children
Medwid, D. and Weston, D.C. (1995)
Clerc Books

Raising and Educating a Deaf Child
Marschark, M. (1997)
Oxford University Press

Internet Resources

▶ www.agbell.org
Information and resources on hearing loss, sensory aids, classroom issues.
Brochures and related books can also be ordered.

▶ www.asha.org
American Speech-Language-Hearing Association. Consumer information
and resources for professionals in speech-language pathology and audiology.

▶ www.jtc.org
The Internet site of the John Tracy Clinic contains contact information for
correspondence courses for parents of children who are deaf and hard of
hearing.

▶ http://clerccenter.gallaudet.edu
Laurent Clerc National Deaf Education Center. Products, training, and
resources related to deafness and hearing loss.

▶ www.nad.org/infocenter
National Association of the Deaf. This Web site addresses legal and
advocacy issues while providing answers to frequently asked questions
regarding deaf culture and ASL.

▶ www. cuedspeech.org
National Cued Speech Association. Information about cued speech,
certification as a cued speech transliterator, and available services for
learning to cue.

▶ www.beginningssvcs.com
Beginnings for Parents of Children Who Are Deaf or Hard-of-Hearing.
An excellent source of information for parents. Topics include early
intervention, communication options, audiology, assistive technology,
and school issues. Many links to related Web sites.

References

Barker, E. J., Dettman, S. J., and Dowell, R. C. (1997). Habilitation: Infants and young children. In G. M. Clark, R. S. Cowan, and R. C. Dowell (Eds.), *Cochlear implantation for infants and children*. San Diego: Singular.

Bebee, H. R., Pearson, H. R., and Koch, M. E. (1984). The Helen Beebe Speech and Hearing Center. In D. Ling (Ed.), *Early intervention for hearing impaired children oral options* (pp. 15-64). Boston: College Hill Press.

Conner, C., Heiber, S., Arts, H., and Zwolan, T. A. (2000). Speech, vocabulary and the education of children using cochlear implants: Oral or total communication? *Journal of Speech-Language and Hearing Research*, 43, 1185-1204.

Cornet, R. O. (1967). Cued speech. *American Annals of the Deaf*, 112, 3-13.

Geers, A. E. (2002). Factors affecting the development of speech, language, and literacy in children with early cochlear implantation. *Language, Speech, and Hearing Services in Schools*, 33, 172-183.

Johnson, R. E., Liddell, S. K., and Erting, C. J. (1990). *Unlocking the curriculum: Principles for achieving access in deaf education*. Washington, D.C.: Gallaudet Research Institute Working Paper 89(3).

Kirk, K. I., Miyamoto, R. T., Ying, E., Perdew, A. E., and Zuganelis, H. (2002). Cochlear implantation in young children: Effects of age at implantation and communication mode. *Volta Review*, 102, 127-144.

Ling, D. (1964). An auditory approach to the education of deaf children. *AuDecibel*, 13, 96-101.

Luetke-Stahlman, B. (1991). Following the rules: Consistency in sign. *Journal of Speech and Hearing Research*, 34, 1293-1298.

Moeller, M. P. (2000). Early intervention and language development in children who are deaf and hard of hearing. *Pediatrics*, 106(3), E43.

Moeller, M. P. and Condon, M. (1998). Family matters: Making sense out of complex issues. In F. Bess (Ed.), *Children with hearing impairments: Contemporary trends*. Nashville, TN: Bill Wilkerson Center Press.

Moeller, M. P., Schick, B., and Williams, K. (1994). *Sign with me*. Omaha, NE: Boystown National Research Hospital.

References, *continued*

Niparko, J., Cheng, A., and Francis, H. (2000). Outcomes of cochlear implantation: Assessment of quality of life impact and evaluation of the benefits of the cochlear implant in relation to costs. In J. Niparko, K. I. Kirk, N. Mellon, A. Robbins, D. Tucci, and B. Wilson (Eds.), *Cochlear implants: Principles and practices.* Philadelphia: Lippincott Williams & Wilkins, Inc.

Osberger, M. J. and Fischer, L. (2000). Preoperative predictors of postoperative implant performance in children. *Annals of Otology, Rhinology, and Laryngology*, 109 (Suppl. 185), 44-46.

Osberger, M. J., Robbins, A., Todd, S., and Riley, A. (1994). Speech intelligibility of children with cochlear implants. *Volta Review*, 96, 169-180.

Paul, P. (2001). *Language and deafness* (3rd ed.). San Diego: Singular Thompson Learning.

Robbins, A. M. (2000). Rehabilitation after implantation. In J. Niparko, K. I. Kirk, N. Mellon, A. Robbins, D. Tucci, and B. Wilson (Eds.), *Cochlear implants: Principles and practices* (pp. 323-363). Philadelphia: Lippincott Williams & Wilkins, Inc.

Ryugo, D. K., Limb, C. J., and Redd, E. E. (2000). Brain plasticity: The impact of environment on the brain as it relates to hearing and deafness. In J. Niparko, K. I. Kirk, N. Mellon, A. Robbins, D. Tucci, and B. Wilson (Eds.), *Cochlear implants: Principles and practices* (pp. 33-56). Philadelphia: Lippincott Williams & Wilkins, Inc.

Schafer, D. and Lynch, J. (1980). Emergent language of six prelingually deaf children. *Teacher of the Deaf*, 5, 94-111.

Schow, R. L. and Nerbonne, M. A. (2002). *Introduction to audiologic rehabilitation* (4th ed.). Boston: Allyn & Bacon.

Scouten, E. (1984). *Turning points in the education of deaf people.* Danville, IL: Interstate Printers and Publishers.

Tobey, E. A., Geers, A. E., Douek, B. M., Perin, J., Skellett, R., and Brenner, C. T. (2000). Factors associated with speech intelligibility in children with cochlear implants. *Annals of Otology, Rhinology & Laryngology*, 109 (Suppl. 185), 28-30.

Vernon, M. and Andrews, J. F. (1990). *The psychology of deafness: Understanding deaf and hard of hearing people.* NY: Longman.

Wilkins, M. and Ertmer, D. J. (2002). Introducing young children who are deaf or hard of hearing to spoken language: Child's Voice, an oral school. *Language, Speech, and Hearing Services in Schools*, 33, 196-204.

Taking Care of Cochlear Implants

5

Parents and professionals share the responsibility for ensuring that young children's cochlear implants work well. The following sections provide basic guidelines for maintaining, checking, and troubleshooting cochlear implants.

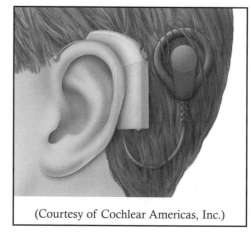

(Courtesy of Cochlear Americas, Inc.)

Cochlear Implant Care

A cochlear implant is an expensive and relatively fragile electronic device. Following a few simple precautions can keep it in good working condition and help to avoid costly repairs.

Handle with care:

▶ Lift and carry the implant without putting stress on the cables.

▶ Don't drop or bang the implant on hard surfaces.

▶ Avoid prolonged exposure to heat, cold, and high humidity.

▶ Treat cables gently; avoid stretching and twisting them.

▶ Electrical shocks can damage speech processors and implant maps. Take the implant off when removing heavy clothing or when the child is playing on plastic playground equipment.

▶ Use a static-reducing product (spray, screen, or floor mat) to reduce the likelihood of shocks around computers and other electronic devices.

▶ Make it a habit to ground yourself by touching metal before handling or removing the child's implant.

▶ Store the implant at room temperature in a place where it is safe from damage from water, pets, or curious children.

▶ Place the implant in a drying kit at night if perspiration or high humidity is a problem.

▶ Never submerge the implant in water. Clean it with a dry cloth.

Daily Visual and Listening Checks

Like any other electronic device, a cochlear implant can malfunction. Performing daily visual and listening checks helps to make "downtime" as short as possible.

Visual Inspections

Visual inspections are usually performed before the speech processor is placed on the child in the morning. Four main steps are involved. First, the speech processor, transmitter, and cables are examined to see whether there are signs of damage (e.g., scratched cases and stretched or worn cables). The microphone port is also inspected to be sure that it is clear of foreign objects. Second, the settings of the device are examined to be sure the proper map, sensitivity, and volume levels are selected. Third, the implant is turned on. Light Emitting Diodes (LEDs) should indicate that the batteries are sufficiently charged. Flashing LEDs and audible alarms may indicate problems with the speech processor or transmitter. Finally, after the implant is in place, a signal wand (provided by the manufacturer) is passed over the transmitter coil to verify that radio waves are being broadcast to the internal receiver. Manufacturer-specific instructions for implant inspections and for interpreting LED and audible alarm signals can be found in user manuals.

Auditory Checks

Next, it is time to check out the quality of the implant signal with an auditory check. The *Ling Six Sound Test* (Ling 1989) is a quick and easy-to-use procedure for estimating how well children detect and perceive speech with their CIs. Parents and clinicians administer this listening check by saying each of the following sounds: /m/, /u/, /a/, /i/, /ʃ/ and /s/, three times in random order at conversational intensity levels. The sounds are presented in a face-to-face situation with the speaker one meter (approximately 3.2 feet) from the child. An acoustic screen (Figure 5.1) is used to cover the mouth so that speechreading cues are concealed. The child is instructed to listen to each speech sound and to either raise a hand

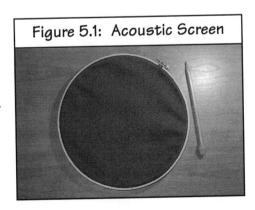

Figure 5.1: Acoustic Screen

when he hears it or repeat it aloud. It is also helpful to remain silent several times during the presentation of Ling sounds so that false positive responses can be detected. The child should respond to silent items by saying/signing "nothing" or shaking his head from side-to-side. The Ling sounds are especially useful because they assess the child's ability to detect and recognize speech sounds across low (/m/ and /u/), mid (/a/ and /i/), and high (/ʃ/ and /s/) frequency ranges.

The first few administrations of the *Ling Six Sound Test* serve as a baseline of the child's initial speech perception abilities with the CI. Increased responsiveness can be expected as the child gains more implant experience. Children who show a persistent decrease in the ability to detect or imitate Ling sounds may be experiencing technological problems. Their audiologists should be contacted if troubleshooting does not result in better performance. Table 5.1 can be used to document children's responses to the Ling sounds. The first row in this table contains an example in which responses are tallied using 1 to denote correct detection/imitation, and 0 to indicate an incorrect response or failure to respond.

Daily visual inspections and listening checks are essential for avoiding long-term equipment breakdowns. Children should also be encouraged to tell parents or teachers about problems or changes in the implant signal as soon as they are noticed. Keeping spare batteries and cables on-hand ensures that the most common technical problems are short-lived.

Table 5.1: A Checklist for Monitoring Ling Sounds (Ling 1989)

Child's name _____ Cochlear implant type _____
Processing strategy _____ Map number _____

Date	/m/	/u/	/a/	/i/	/ʃ/	/s/
Ex: 1/25/05	111	111	111	110	111	001

Comments _____
_____
_____
_____

Troubleshooting

Troubleshooting is the process of determining what is broken and how the problem can be fixed. Some implant breakdowns have simple solutions that parents and professionals can implement. These include replacing batteries and cords or cleaning battery contacts. Other problems may require shipping the implant to a repair center. In the latter case, a loaner speech processor is often supplied by the center or the manufacturer.

Troubleshooting procedures vary according to each type of CI. Lists of common problems and solutions can be found in user manuals and at the Web sites listed below. Professionals and parents should familiarize themselves with these resources ahead of time so that implant malfunctions can be remedied as soon as possible.

▶ Advanced Bionics Corporation
   www.bcig.org/contact/manufa.htm#advanced

▶ Cochlear Corporation
   www.cochlearamericas.com/recipients/149.asp

▶ Med-El Corporation
   www.medel.com (search for "daily checks")

▶ The Listening Center at Johns Hopkins
   www.thelisteningcenter.com

▶ The Family Support Connection of Minnesota
   www.familysupportconnection.org/index.htm

Now that the reader is familiar with cochlear implant technology, candidacy requirements, communication modalities, and the services that are provided soon after surgery, it is time to consider clinical approaches to developing communication skills in children with CIs. The second half of this book will address this topic for infants and toddlers, preschoolers, and school-age children.

Reference

Ling, D. (1989). *Foundation of spoken language for hearing-impaired children.* Washington, D.C.: A.G. Bell Association.

Introduction to Part 2
Communication Intervention for Children with Cochlear Implants

The second part of this book offers a variety of approaches for helping children with CIs maximize their oral communication abilities. This information is presented for three age groups: infants and toddlers (Chapter 6), preschoolers (Chapter 7), and school-age children (Chapter 8). In cases where the content of these chapters can be applied to more than one age group, the overlap will be noted in the affected chapters. The approaches offered in these chapters are drawn from the research and clinical literatures for children with hearing loss and children with normal hearing who have speech and language disorders. As such, they represent currently accepted practices more than the results of treatment efficacy studies. The ideas in the following chapters are intended for implanted children who use oral or signed forms of communication and, in many cases, can also be applied to children who have mild-severe hearing losses and wear hearing aids. A few definitions are helpful before going further.

Aural rehabilitation has been defined as "intervention aimed at minimizing and alleviating the communication difficulties associated with hearing loss" (Tye-Murray 1998, p. 2). These difficulties fall into three main categories: listening, speaking, and oral language. The content of the upcoming chapters will focus on ways to increase competence in each of these areas. A second term, *aural habilitation*, refers specifically to treatment programs for children with prelingual hearing loss. This term is needed because most children with an early onset of hearing loss must develop new skills—rather than recover lost abilities—with their CIs. In order to discuss services for children with cochlear implants in a cohesive way, we will use the term *communication intervention* for activities encompassed in auditory re/habilitation programs for children with CIs.

Communication intervention can be implemented by SLPs, teachers of children with hearing loss, or audiologists. In recognition of the involvement of each of these professions, the terms *interventionist* and *clinician* will be used to refer to the professionals who are charged with developing and implementing communication intervention programs. *Early Interventionist* (EI) will be used for those who work with the families of infants and toddlers with hearing loss.

Main Components of Communication Intervention

Communication intervention programs consist of three main elements: counseling, communication assessment, and intervention. Each component is essential for optimizing children's oral communication abilities.

Counseling

Counseling takes many forms in aural habilitation programs. For infants and toddlers who have CIs, counseling focuses on helping parents recognize opportunities to stimulate listening, speech, and language during everyday interactions. It is also used to support parents as they develop a realistic understanding of the effects of hearing loss on spoken language development and the special needs of their children. A broader approach to counseling is needed as children enter school settings.

Throughout the child's educational career, interventionists continue to interact with parents while also assuming increased responsibility for counseling classroom teachers. The latter form of counseling involves providing information about hearing loss and CIs, answering technology-related questions, suggesting ways to optimize the listening environment (see Chapter 9), and identifying and addressing curricular and communication needs, among many other topics. Effective interventionists also pay attention to the emotional needs of the child and attempt to facilitate positive transitions into new social and educational situations. Counseling is a dynamic and on-going process that is crucial for the success of an aural habilitation program. Suggestions for effective counseling will be made in each of the next three chapters.

Communication Assessments

Communication assessments are chosen according to the age and the skill level of the child. For infants and toddlers, the benefits of implantation may be most reliably examined by observing reactions to sounds and speech, by listening for changes in the kinds of vocalizations that the child produces, or by noticing when words are comprehended and produced. As children enter preschool, their communication skills can also be examined through the use of formal tests and criterion-referenced tasks. A mix of standardized tests, language samples, and criterion-referenced tasks is commonly used to examine communication ability in school-age children. In addition, adolescents and young adults may be able to evaluate some of their own communicative behaviors and select personally relevant goals. Chapters 6–8 contain specific suggestions for assessing oral communication skills with age-appropriate tools.

Communication Intervention

Communication intervention models also change as children grow older and become better communicators. Parents are the natural choice for stimulating listening, speech, and language development in infants and toddlers because they have abundant opportunities for interacting with their child. Interventionists take advantage of parent-child closeness by employing a family-centered approach to aural habilitation during this time. This approach continues to be useful as children enter preschool and begin to receive clinician-directed as well as child-centered intervention. Interventionists and classroom teachers gain increasing responsibility for communication development as children enter elementary school. The importance of oral language abilities for academic success cannot be overemphasized during this time. Intervention models that address both developmental language and functional communication needs can go a long way toward helping children achieve academic and social success. Whereas no single intervention model is a perfect fit for every child, the upcoming chapters provide a variety of useful strategies for clinicians to consider. It is expected that skillful interventionists will modify them to meet the individual communication needs of the children and families they serve.

Classroom Acoustics and Future Developments

The classroom listening environment has a large impact on communicative and academic success for preschool and school-age children with CIs. Chapter 9 explores factors that influence the quality of the speech signal in the classroom as well as ways to improve classroom acoustics so that children can make the most of their implants or hearing aids. Finally, Chapter 10 provides a look to the future by considering some imminent and some long-range advancements in implant technology, and by identifying areas for future improvements in clinical service provision.

Reference

Tye-Murray, N. M. (1998). *Foundation of aural rehabilitation.* San Diego: Singular Publishing.

Family-Centered Intervention for Infants and Toddlers with CIs

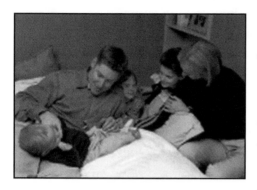

The importance of early identification and intervention for infants with hearing losses has been clearly confirmed by two recent research studies. These studies have direct implications for providing communication intervention for very young cochlear implant recipients. In the first investigation, Yoshinaga-Itano et al. (1998) examined the language abilities of children whose hearing losses were identified either before six months of age or after that time. The children in both groups began to receive intervention services within two months after identification, on average. Follow-up testing revealed that children whose hearing losses were identified by six months of age had acquired significantly better language abilities than those who were identified after six months of age. This advantage was noted across all ages, communication modalities, socioeconomic levels, and degrees of hearing loss. No additional variables (besides age-at-identification) appeared to account for the difference between the two groups. The findings of this study have provided solid support for Universal Newborn Hearing Screening (UNHS) programs.

It has also been shown that the age at which young children with hearing loss begin to receive intervention is predictive of later language abilities. Moeller (2000) examined the relationship between the age at enrollment in intervention programs and the language skills of five-year-old children who were deaf or hard of hearing. She found that children who were enrolled in intervention programs before 11 months of age had developed larger vocabularies and better verbal reasoning skills than those who first received services after that age. Further examination of the factors that influenced language development revealed that family involvement was highly correlated with achievement levels. That is, children with better language skills were likely to have parents who were active participants in the intervention process. The most successful children in this study were those who had been enrolled in intervention by 11 months and who had high levels of family involvement. Referencing the Yoshinaga-Itano study, Moeller concluded that "success is achieved when early identification is paired with early interventions that actively involve families."

Recognition of the importance of early identification and intervention has led to the implementation of UNHS, PL 94-457, and the Individuals with Disabilities Education Act (IDEA). Regulations for the latter legislation also emphasize the value of family involvement by shifting the focus of the early intervention efforts from the child to the family. That is, rather than concentrating primarily on the communicative needs of the child (i.e., a child-centered approach), Early Interventionists (EIs) are now encouraged to help parents develop nurturing and responsive relationships with their children through a family-centered approach to service provision.

Family-Centered Intervention

Family-centered intervention recognizes the crucial roles that parents play in helping infants and toddlers reach their communication potentials (Donahue-Kilburg 1992, Rossetti 2001). Using this approach, parents are viewed as partners with EIs, and their opinions and input are considered essential for the development of an Individual Family Service Plan (IFSP). Such a collaborative relationship develops over time as the family's values, expectations, and priorities are shared with, and respected by, the interventionist. Thus, parents of children with CIs should be supported, rather than directed, as they learn to provide auditory, speech, and language stimulation throughout the day. This support takes many forms.

The family is supported when EIs thoughtfully consider parents' observations, concerns, and cultural perspectives about their child. By recognizing parents as experts on their own child, the interventionist empowers them to become actively involved in important processes such as choosing a communication modality, selecting intervention priorities, and monitoring progress. EIs also provide support by highlighting the skills and knowledge that parents already possess. Acknowledging parents' interaction strengths can help to increase confidence and reduce stress. It is important to remember, however, that parents differ in their readiness to participate in family-centered intervention.

Some parents seem to have a knack for helping their children learn to communicate. They easily play at the child's level, initiate turn-taking and take advantage of incidental learning opportunities. Other parents may be unsure of how to communicate with a child who has a hearing loss. Still others may be inclined to let you, "the expert," work with the child while they take a break or deal with pressing household matters. All parents have some interaction strengths, however.

These strengths may be as basic as willingness to hold and rock the child when sleepy, to talk to the baby during meals, or to return a toy that has been dropped. Finding and reinforcing each parent's interaction strengths is an important step toward an effective partnership.

Offering choices can also help parents view themselves as active partners in the intervention process. For example, some parents may wish to observe EI-child interactions before trying out language stimulation techniques. Others may want to read related materials and discuss ideas before adopting them. Still others may ask for "on-line" coaching as they try out new strategies. Supporting personal preferences allows parents to see themselves as respected partners in their child's program. This perception is reinforced as EIs and parents interact in a flexible, patient, and positive way.

Six parent-child interaction enhancement techniques should be discussed with parents during the early stages of intervention (see Table 6.1). Each technique increases the likelihood that attempts to stimulate listening, speech, and language development will be effective. These techniques may be best introduced through demonstrations, followed by coaching and positive feedback as parents attempt to modify their interaction styles accordingly. It is often advisable to introduce a few techniques at a time.

Table 6.1: Interaction Enhancement Techniques	
1. Establish Joint Attention	• Position yourself at the child's eye level during interactions and play. • Focus your attention on what the child is doing, listening to, or looking at. Resist the urge to control his attention. Follow the child's lead by commenting on his interests.
2. Encourage Turn-taking	• Initiate give-and-take during physical play, quiet play, and book reading by encouraging the child to respond and waiting for a response expectantly. • Remember to share control of your "conversations" by pausing and allowing the child to initiate communication.
3. Respond to Nonverbal Communication Cues and Vocalizations	• Your child's speech, gestures, facial expressions, and eye gaze can communicate thoughts, feelings, and desires. React to nonverbal cues and vocalizations by giving the child a desired object, saying a related response, or acting puzzled if you don't understand.
4. Establish Communication Routines Throughout the Day	• Describe everyday tasks such as dressing, feeding, and getting ready for bed as you do them. Repeat selected vocabulary words multiple times during each routine. • Play with the same toys using the same vocabulary to describe the toys and their actions.
5. Make Everyday Sounds Meaningful	• Let the child know whenever you hear new environmental sounds. Saying "I hear that" or "I hear (someone)" while pointing to your ear can help the child alert to sounds and associate them with their sources. • Have something new or interesting to give/show whenever you call the child's name.
6. Make Your Speech Easier to Understand	• Speak at a slightly slower rate. • Speak slightly louder than normal. • Vary intonation patterns. • Use gestures and facial expressions when speaking. • Emphasize key words.

Stimulating Listening, Language, and Speech Development

Young CI recipients have the important advantage of beginning to hear within an age-range when many foundational speech and language skills are typically acquired. This "early" start, when combined with effective intervention, can help them to acquire auditory skills at a near-normal rate (Robbins et al. 2003). It is important to remember, however, that children with CIs do not have normal hearing ability. Their aided thresholds commonly range between 20 and 40 dB HL across the speech frequencies. Reduced sound localization ability (due to unilateral rather than bilateral hearing) and excessive background noise also impact spoken language development negatively. Specialized intervention strategies are needed to reduce the adverse effects of these ongoing problems.

The following sections provide suggestions for assessing and optimizing auditory, speech, and oral language development in infants and toddlers who have CIs. Although these elements of communication are discussed separately, it is recognized that they are fully integrated in meaningful communication and during most language stimulation activities. These recommendations are based on recently proposed strategies for children with CIs, on intervention frameworks developed for normally hearing children with communication disorders, and on the acoustic characteristics of speech. As such, they represent accepted clinical practices to a greater extent than the findings of intervention efficacy studies. Clinicians are encouraged to modify suggested activities and intervention frameworks, as needed, to meet the needs of the individuals they serve.

Assessing Auditory Abilities

EIs typically spend one hour per week with each family they serve. Thus, the great majority of the child's development occurs during the remaining 167 hours of the week. A diary is a helpful way for parents to keep track of changes in listening, speech, and oral language behaviors during this time. Diaries can take many forms. For some parents, they might consist of a few, brief entries that list new speech sounds or words. Other parents may use diaries to document a wide variety of listening and social behaviors along with detailed interpretations of these situations. Some parents may find that their busy schedules do not allow them to make written diary entries and may prefer to remember behaviors rather than write them down.

In each of these cases, it is important to discuss key distinctions in communication behaviors so that behaviors can be described accurately.

The difference between imitative and spontaneous behaviors is well-understood by communication professionals, but might not be readily apparent to parents. EIs may need to ask parents to describe their observations in greater detail when the context of an observation is not clear. For example, a parent may report that the child said "dog" one day. The EI's simple request to "Tell me about the time Jimmy said 'dog,' " may reveal that his older sister elicited his production by modeling it several times and telling Jimmy to say it. It may also become apparent that his production was actually an isolated /ɔ/ rather than [dɔg]. Finally, it might be the case that Jimmy said "dog" after the family pet was out of sight. Thus, saying "dog" didn't necessarily mean that he understood the word. A clear understanding of the distinctions between imitative and spontaneous productions, between comprehension and expression, and between the child's actual spoken utterance and the adult-like speech target is necessary for parents to accurately describe their child's communicative behaviors.

In addition to direct observation and examination of diary entries, EIs will find a structured interview very helpful in gaining a comprehensive picture of post-implantation progress. *The Infant-Toddler Meaningful Auditory Integration Scale* (*IT-MAIS*, Zimmerman-Phillips et al. 1997) is a parent interview tool that consists of ten questions that focus on auditory and speech development. Administering the *IT-MAIS* prior to, or soon after implantation, can provide a baseline for comparison with performance at three- or six-month intervals. Robbins (2003) has compiled a valuable collection of intervention strategies for each *IT-MAIS* item. These ideas can be especially useful in selecting and working toward communication goals.

Parents are in an ideal position to notice changes in auditory, speech, and language behaviors. They see their children in a wide variety of situations that may elicit new responses to sounds and new forms of self-expression. Although parents have the opportunity to witness these events, they often need help in identifying key, auditory-based behaviors. One of the essential roles of the EI is to help parents recognize changes in their child's communicative abilities. Table 6.2 on page 78 contains a list of early emerging auditory behaviors that can indicate improved auditory perception following implantation. EIs can use this table to determine how frequently a selected behavior is observed (i.e., Sometimes, Often, Not Observed) based on repeated parent reports during the first year of CI experience.

Table 6.2: An Informal Rating Scale of Early Emerging Auditory and Speech Behaviors in Infants and Toddlers with Cochlear Implants

Directions: Enter the date of each rating and either **S = Sometimes**, **O = Often**, or **NO = Not Observed** in the boxes below. Information is gathered from parent report.

Child's name _____   Age at implantation _____

Parent's name _____   Clinician _____

Behavior	Time 1	Time 2	Time 3	Time 4	Comments
1. Wears CI without resistance					
2. Reacts to loud sounds in the environment					
3. Explores the sound-making capabilities of common objects and toys					
4. Responds to loud speech					
5. Looks at people when they are talking					
6. Vocalizes "back and forth" with other talkers					
7. Looks for the source of environmental sounds					
8. Reacts to medium or soft environmental sounds					
9. Pays attention to singing, humming, or music					
10. Associates sounds with their sources (e.g., telephone, microwave oven signals)					
11. Turns when name is called					
12. Attends to speech or singing for several minutes					
13. Understands single words					
14. Repeats single words or short phrases					
15. Listens attentively to speech during book reading					

Facilitating Auditory Development

For infants with normal hearing, auditory skills are developed in a self-directed manner as sound becomes associated with meaning. That is, once children realize that environmental sounds have predictable sources and that speech represents concepts that can be personally important, they actively search for the meanings of sounds (Ling and Ling 1978). Infants and toddlers with CIs typically require special help to detect, discriminate, identify, and comprehend the sounds they hear. In addition to the six interaction enhancement techniques described on page 75, parents and EIs can provide a variety of experiences that will help children associate sound with meaning. These involve exposure to both environmental sounds and speech.

Opportunities to improve detection and identification of environmental sounds are available throughout the day. By modeling a *hearing response* (e.g., saying "I hear that" while pointing to your ear) parents can help children become aware of telephone rings, microwave buzzers, doorbells, and other audible signals around the house. Outdoor sounds such as birds singing, car horns, dogs barking, and cheering at sports events also provide opportunities for modeling a hearing response.   In each case, parents should look at the child expectantly after modeling a hearing response and repeat the model while the sound continues to be heard. Eventually, children should begin to respond to sounds by pointing to their ears. Spontaneous alerting to sound should be encouraged and celebrated whenever it occurs so that the value of listening becomes apparent to the child.

Most parents engage in vocal play and one-sided "conversations" with infants from the moment they are born. They pretend that the child can actually understand what is being said and that the child's gestures and vocalizations have clear meaning. This sort of "linguistic bath" is also very important for helping young implant recipients become aware of the nature of speech and the meanings of words. In addition to talking during routine activities, parents can stimulate speech perception as they play with their child. Games that involve turn-taking and repeated phrases are especially appropriate during the first months of implant experience. Examples of these include playing Peek-a-Boo; saying "up, up, up" and "down, down, down" as the child is lifted repeatedly; playing with a jack-in-the-box; and riding a "horse" as the parent "neighs."

Parents also encounter many *teachable moments* for stimulating speech perception and language development. These opportunities arise spontaneously as children become actively interested in the objects and events around them. Parents can take advantage of these learning opportunities by sharing the child's interest and then providing related comments. For example, the child may find a worm on the sidewalk. By overtly looking at the worm and making a comment or two (e.g., "Worm. Worms live in dirt."), the child is given the opportunity to "tie" sound to meaning in a naturally intriguing context. Teachable moments occur throughout the day and are especially helpful for developing an understanding of the world and expanding vocabulary.

Assessing Language Skills

Because of their greatly increased potential for auditory learning and relatively young age at implantation, typical patterns of language development should serve as a guide for stimulating and monitoring the acquisition of spoken language skills in young CI users. Key linguistic milestones for typically developing children include true comprehension of single words (~9-12 months), first spoken words (~1 year), and first-word combinations (~18-24 months). Progress toward these milestones is usually assessed by observing the child during everyday situations. This informal approach is needed because very young children are not able to consistently attend to structured tasks, follow directions, or respond "on command" as required in formal testing situations. Thus, both parents and clinicians need to monitor the emergence of new receptive and expressive language behaviors to estimate post-implantation progress. Although it has been shown that some children can successfully participate in structured testing after 30 months of age (Robbins and Kirk 1996), our discussion of assessment procedures will focus on ways to document progress in auditory and spoken language development through observation and interviews.

The Communication Development Inventory (*CDI*; Fenson et al. 1993) is commonly used to measure receptive and expressive vocabulary growth after cochlear implantation. There are two forms of this parent report. The Words and Gestures form is most appropriate for monitoring growth in non-verbal communication and single word vocabulary. It should be given during the first-word period of language development (8–16 months in children with normal hearing). The Words and Sentences form examines single word vocabulary, word combinations, and grammatical morphemes and it was developed for children between 16 and 30 months of age. Each of these checklists requires parents to identify vocabulary words and constructions that their child understands and/or produces spontaneously.

Administering the *CDI* soon after the child begins to say words, and at six-month intervals thereafter, will allow parents and EIs to determine the rate at which new words, word combinations, and grammatical constructions appear. The child's expressive vocabulary should also increase in the variety of word classes so that nouns, verbs, adjectives, and prepositions become represented. It is important to remember that norms for the *CDI* were developed with children who hear normally. Children with CIs will have smaller vocabularies than their age peers as they learn to comprehend the implant signal and express themselves.

Children's two- and three-word combinations can provide evidence that they are acquiring greater facility with language. The use of semantic relations such as negation (e.g., "no milk"), possession (e.g., "Daddy car"), location (e.g., "Mommy gone"), agent-action (e.g., "Baby cry") indicate the child has developed the ability to express more complex ideas. Similarly, careful attention should be paid to whether the child is using language for a variety of purposes. These include, but are not limited to, making statements and asking questions. Traditional sampling measures of language ability such as *Type-Token Ratio* (Templin 1957) and *Mean Length of Utterance* (Brown 1973) can be completed as children begin to use word combinations and sentences on a regular basis.

Auditory comprehension is difficult to measure through observation unless the directions are given without accompanying nonverbal cues (e.g., gestures, pointing, or limited choices for responding). The ability to follow progressively longer spoken directions (e.g., "Give me ball" or "Bring your shoes and socks"), however, provides an indication that auditory comprehension ability is increasing. In summary, progress in acquiring early emerging receptive and expressive language skills can be monitored with many of the same observational tools used with infants and toddlers who have normal hearing.

Facilitating Language Development

Leonard (1992) has described a variety of input, response, and clarification strategies that are commonly used to stimulate language development in children with Specific Language Impairment (SLI; see Tables 6.3 and 6.4 on pages 83 and 84 respectively). Because children with CIs appear to acquire language skills in a near-typical sequence (Brackett and Zara 1998), these techniques have the potential to be useful for this population as well. Input strategies expose children to language models that are similar to or slightly more advanced than those they already produce. For example, if the child does not say any words, parents and clinicians make an effort to use many single word utterances when talking to the child. Response strategies build on what the child has just said by acknowledging, responding to, or modifying the child's utterance. Clarification strategies are used by adults when a child utterance is not understood.

Introducing these strategies judiciously can help parents develop their language stimulation skills without being overwhelmed by the number of different techniques available.

Table 6.3: Language Input Strategies	
1. Speak in a slightly slower than normal rate and articulate clearly.	12. Repeat key words several times and emphasize them over other words. (Focused stimulation)
2. Communicate face-to-face and at the child's level whenever possible.	13. Encourage the child to use words or phrases in appropriate situations (e.g., "Say 'wake up'"). (Coaching)
3. Use utterances that are the same length or slightly longer than the child's usual utterances.	14. Rephrase adult utterances by decreasing the number of words. For example, change "I want to go home" to "Want go home." (Breakdowns)
4. Repeat messages several times.	
5. Use gestures, facial expressions, and body language to accompany messages.	15. Rephrase simple adult utterances by adding elements. For example, first say, "Bath time" and then "It's time for your bath." (Build-ups)
6. Use consistent labels for items until the child understands or produces the word. Then begin to introduce synonyms. For example, use *coat* at first and then introduce *jacket*.	
	16. Pause frequently so that the child can process information and take a conversational turn.
7. Vary intonation and loudness to emphasize specific words.	17. Use choice, open-ended, or rhetorical questions rather than questions that require a "yes/no" answer. For example, ask, "Do you want juice or milk?" or say, "I wonder who's at the door."
8. Describe the on-going action and interests of the child. (Parallel talk)	
9. Describe your actions and interests. (Self-talk)	
10. Provide words for your child's wants, feelings, and intended messages.	18. Provide the answer to your questions at the child's level if he does not respond after a few moments. For example, ask, "Do you want grape or strawberry?" If he doesn't answer, say, "Oh, you want grape."
11. Model words and phrases that are related to what the child is looking at or doing.	

(Adapted from Leonard, J. S. [1992]. Communication intervention for children at risk for specific communication disorders. *Seminars in Speech and Language*, 13, 223-235. Reprinted by permission.)

Table 6.4: Response and Clarification Strategies	
Response Strategies (what to say after the child talks)	**Clarification Strategies** (what to do when the child can't be understood)
1. Repeat the child's utterances to affirm the message.	1. Repeat any part of the child's message that is understood. For example, say, "Daddy? What about Daddy?"
2. Repeat the child's utterance, adding one or two new elements. For example, the child says, "car." The adult responds, "Fast car!" or "Mommy's car" depending on the child's interest.	2. Ask choice questions to clarify the child's messages. For example, ask, "Did you say 'See bus' or 'Stop bus'?"
3. Repeat elements of the child's utterance in a different construction. For example, the child says, "Mommy purse." The adult responds, "Where's Mommy's purse?"	3. Ask the child to show you what he wants. Pointing and gestures can provide clues to the child's meaning and offer opportunities to model language.
4. Recognize and restate the child's messages even if the intent is undesirable. For example, say, "You want cookie. No, no cookie now."	4. Remember the child's speech patterns and use them to help you understand unintelligible messages. For example, if the child says "t" for "s," then his production of "ti" for "see" will be understood more easily.
5. Provide words to express the child's feelings even if they are unpleasant. For example, if the child protests leaving a friend's house by crying, the adult can say, "No. No go. Don't want to go."	5. Know the topics that interest your child so that you can more easily figure out what he is saying.
6. Highlight new speech sounds and words as they emerge in the child's repertoire.	6. Acknowledge frustration. It can be helpful to take the blame for the communication breakdown. For example, say, "I'm sorry, I don't understand. We'll try later."
7. Contrast immature and more adult-like utterances. For example, say, "Wawa? Oh, you want water."	7. Model self-corrections occasionally. For example, say, "Go get your tocks. Oh, I mean socks."
(Adapted from Leonard, J. S. [1992]. Communication intervention for children at risk for specific communication disorders. *Seminars in Speech and Language*, 13, 223-235. Reprinted by permission.)	

Assessing Vocal Development

(Portions of this section adapted from Ertmer, Young, et al. [2002] and used with permission of the American Speech-Language-Hearing Association)

Vocal development is the process by which children begin to produce increasingly complex, phonetically diverse, and speech-like utterances before they say words on a regular basis. The nature of vocal development in children with cochlear implants can best be understood through comparison with typically developing and hearing-impaired children. Typically-developing infants produce increasingly more complex and speech-like vocalizations during their first two years of life (Oller 1980, Stark 1980, Vihman 1996). These gains are generally recognized as the foundation for meaningful speech because the vowels, consonants, and syllable shapes found in later prelinguistic vocalizations are also common in a child's first words (Vihman et al. 1986). Research has shown that hearing loss has a negative impact on vocal development.

There are several notable differences in the vocal development of deaf and normally hearing infants and toddlers. In general, the prelinguistic speech of deaf toddlers is characterized by a delayed onset of babbling (Oller and Eilers 1988), restricted formant frequency range (Kent et al. 1987), reduced phonetic and syllabic inventories (Stoel-Gammon and Otomo 1986), relatively greater final syllable lengthening (Nathani et al. 2002), and an absence of expressive jargon and prewords (Stark 1983). Deficits in these areas may contribute to limitations in later phonological development in young hearing-impaired children (Ertmer and Stark 1995). Because of their relatively greater aided hearing sensitivity, young children with CIs can be expected to make gains in vocal development beyond those noted for deaf toddlers who use hearing aids.

In addition to responding to environmental sounds and speech in a meaningful way (e.g., searching for a ringing telephone, turning when their names are called), young implant recipients should begin to produce well-formed and speech-like vocalizations as they are exposed to mature speech patterns and auditory feedback (Ertmer et al. 2002, Ertmer and Mellon 2001, McCaffrey et al. 1999). Understanding the course of vocal development can enable EIs to document progress in speech development and stimulate speech skills before children begin to say words on a regular basis.

A three-level classification system has been proposed by Ertmer and colleagues to describe vocal development in children who receive CIs before their third birthdays (Ertmer and Mellon 2001, Ertmer et al. 2002). This approach is a consolidation of the five-level system used in the *Stark Assessment of Early Vocal Development-Revised* (*SAEVD-R*; Nathani et al. 2002). Table 6.5 contains descriptions of vocalizations at three successive levels: Precanonical, Canonical Syllables, and Advanced Forms (also called "postcanonical" in Ertmer and Mellon 2001). It is recommended that EIs visit www.vocaldevelopment.com (Ertmer and Galster 2001) to listen to examples of each vocalization type and to complete a self-test before attempting to classify children's utterances. Further guidelines for classifying utterances and a document for classifying utterances are provided in Table 6.6 on page 88.

The following criteria have been found to be useful indicators of progress in vocal development in children who were implanted before their third birthdays (Ertmer, Young, and Nathani, manuscript in preparation).

1) Canonical Syllable utterances comprise ≥ 20% of two consecutive samples (if the child had not reached this level before implantation)

2) Advanced Form utterances comprise ≥ 20% of two consecutive samples

3) Precanonical utterances are less frequently produced than those from the Canonical Syllables and Advanced Form levels

The rate at which young implant recipients typically achieve the above milestones in vocal development is currently being investigated.

Chapter 6: Family-Centered Intervention for Infants and Toddlers with CIs

Table 6.5: Levels of Vocal Development

	Precanonical Vocalizations* Typical age of emergence: 0 - 6 months	Canonical Syllables* Typical age of emergence: 6 - 10 months	Advanced Forms/Postcanonical* Approximate age of emergence: 10 - 18 months
Description	Vocalizations lack true vowels and true consonants in combination with a rapid transition between them	Vocalizations characterized by: 1. Normal phonation 2. At least one consonant and one vowel in combination 3. Rapid transition between consonant and vowel (Oller and Lynch 1992)	Vocalizations have the characteristics of Canonical Syllables but are more complex and later-emerging in typically developing children (Nathani, Ertmer, and Stark 2002)
Examples	1. Squeals 2. Grunts 3. Vowel-like sounds in isolation 4. Multiple vowel-like sounds in a series 5. Closants sounds such as clicks, lip smacks, or "raspberries" 6. Isolated consonants (e.g., /m/, /n/)	1. CV syllables 2. CVCV syllables 3. Rhythmic production of reduplicated babbling (e.g., babababa) 4. Rhythmic production of non-reduplicated babbling (e.g., didapa) 5. Whispered vocalizations	1. Closed syllables (e.g., CVC) 2. Consonant clusters (e.g, CCV) 3. Jargon (i.e., syllable strings with different vowels and consonants overlaid with rhythmic stress, intonation changes, or both)

* Audio examples of three types of vocalizations can be heard at www.vocaldevelopment.com (Ertmer and Galster 2001).
(Adapted from Ertmer et al. 2002, Nathani et al. 2002)

Table 6.6: Rules for Classifying Utterances into Levels of Vocal Development

▲ Classify 50 spontaneous or imitative utterances as either precanonical, canonical syllables, or advanced forms.

▲ An utterance is a vocalization or group of vocalizations separated from others by ≥ 1 second or ingressive breath.

▲ Classify only speech-related vocalizations. Do not include coughs, cries, screams, laughs, snorts, or burps, etc.

▲ Do not count /h/ as a consonant.

▲ Count glides (/j/ or /w/) as true consonants only if they are combined with vowels at a near normal rate (i.e., not slowly).

▲ Classify each utterance according to its most developmentally advanced component (e.g., if an utterance contains a series of vowels, reduplicated babbling, and a squeal, the entire utterance would be classified at the Canonical Syllable level because of the reduplicated babbling.)

▲ Each level can be considered "established" when it accounts for at least 20% of the child's vocalizations.

Form for estimating level of vocal development

Date	Precanonical	Canonical Syllables	Advanced Forms
May 14, 2004	11111 11111 11111 11111 11111 = 25/50 (50%)	11111 11111 11111 11111 = 20/50 (40%)	11111 = 5/50 (10%)

Facilitating Vocal Development

Although the mechanisms of vocal learning in young children are not well understood, imitation and social interaction appear to play key roles in early development. For example, in an investigation of vowel imitation, Kuhl and Meltzoff (1996) showed that normally hearing infants at 12, 16, and 20 weeks produced /u/, /i/, and /a/ more frequently while listening and watching videotapes of an adult saying the same vowels repeatedly. The authors concluded that "A total of 15 minutes of exposure (i.e., five minutes of exposure to a specific vowel on each of three days) was sufficient to influence vocalizations in infants under 20 weeks of age" (p. 2435). Although imitation of a variety of speech patterns and sounds was not examined, these findings show that concentrated modeling can influence vocalizations in typically-developing infants. They also suggest that this technique may be useful for stimulating speech development in young children with cochlear implants.

Short Periods of Prelinguistic Input (SPPI, Ertmer et al. 2002) is an intervention approach that is intended to stimulate vocal development through concentrated modeling. The aim of SPPI is to help children progress from the Precanonical to the Canonical Syllables and to the Advanced Forms levels so that they acquire a base of prelinguistic speech skills for phonological and lexical development. This goal is addressed by providing repeated models of prelinguistic vocalizations and reinforcing the child's imitative attempts. SPPI can be used in remediation with children who show delays in vocal development, or as a systematic way to stimulate auditory perception and vocal development in newly-implanted children. In both cases, parents and clinicians provide models of vocalizations from the child's current level of development before emphasizing vocalizations from progressively higher levels. This approach has face validity because it applies modeling, a well-accepted instructional method in the early stages of speech and language intervention (Bernthal and Bankson 1988, Leonard 1992), to stimulate speech skills in a progression similar to that observed in typically developing infants and toddlers (see Oller 2000, Vihman 1996 for reviews). SPPI is intended to supplement previously described strategies for stimulating auditory and language skills.

SPPI Procedures

Kuhl and Meltzoff (1996) used videotape recordings of an adult producing a target vowel every five seconds for five minutes to stimulate vowel production in infants. While this amount of modeling effectively influenced vocalizations, few parents or clinicians could tolerate repeating the same vocalization for this length of time. A more viable alternative is to provide one-minute periods of *concentrated modeling* during vocal play exchanges several times daily. Although the optimal number of modeling periods per day is unknown, providing SPPI at least five times per day ensures a match with the procedures of the Kuhl and Meltzoff study. Models of the target vocalization are presented at a rate of approximately one vocalization every five seconds (12 vocalizations per minute), allowing an opportunity for imitation during the pauses between models.

Targets for modeling are selected according to the child's observed level of vocal development (i.e., the highest level that comprises 20% of all utterances). In this way, a variety of vocalizations within the child's developmental ability are reinforced and expanded before higher-level vocalization types are introduced. For example, initial targets for newly implanted children and those who produce few canonical syllables would include a wide range of vowel sounds. The methods used in the Kuhl and Meltzoff study suggest an initial emphasis on point vowels (i.e., /i/, /a/, /u/, and /æ/) may be beneficial possibly due to the highly salient acoustic differences between these targets. Other vowels can be introduced as the child begins to imitate and spontaneously produce point vowels.

As the child begins to imitate and spontaneously produce a variety of vowels more freely, canonical syllables can be highlighted through repeated models of CV syllables, disyllables (CVCV), and reduplicated and non-reduplicated syllable strings. Modeling visibly salient consonants (e.g., /p/, /b/, /m/, /w/) may help children associate sounds with articulator movements at first. Combining visible consonants with vowels that the child already produces provides an opportunity to build new phonetic combinations from those that have been learned previously. Consonants with different place, manner, and voicing features can be targeted as the child begins to imitate or spontaneously produce syllables with visible consonants. Newly targeted consonants are also combined with a variety of vowels. As Yoshinaga-Itano (2000) notes, including models of high frequency consonants along with low- and mid-frequency phonemes ensures that the auditory nerve is stimulated for the full spectrum of speech sounds.

Advanced Forms can be introduced after the child readily imitates a variety of canonical syllables with different vowel and consonant combinations or begins to produce more advanced forms spontaneously. In particular, VC and CVC syllables and jargon should be emphasized to expand the child's syllable shape inventory and increase the use of varied intonation and stress patterns.

Finally, SPPI should be provided within the context of vocal play and during interactions that are calm and mutually enjoyable. The auditory and visual saliency of the models can be enhanced by speaking slightly louder than normal and by facing the child whenever possible. Variations in intonation and rhythm are also important for encouraging imitation and stimulating control of suprasegmental speech features. Although models of vocalizations can be presented by themselves, they may be more interesting when associated with toys and actions as suggested by Estabrooks (1998). For example, "bababa" can be paired with a sheep and /aʊ/ ("ow") with a pretend injury. The use of toys may also encourage turn-taking. More information about SPPI and video examples of concentrated modeling can be found at www.vocaldevelopment.com (Ertmer and Galster 2001).

Identifying Insufficient Progress After Implantation

Robbins (2003) has identified six warning signs of inadequate progress (see Table 6.7 below) in young children with CIs. Parents and EIs should be aware of these red flags and discuss any concerns with the child's implant team.

Table 6.7: Warning Signs of Inadequate Progress

1. Full-time use not accomplished one month after initial stimulation

2. No change in the quality or quantity of vocalizations after three months of device use

3. Skills demonstrated in audiological testing not observed in everyday settings

4. Child not spontaneously alerting to own name after six months of device use

5. Lack of spontaneous alerting to environmental sounds six months after hook-up

6. No evidence of meaning being derived from sound after 12 months of device use

(Robbins 2003, p. 22)

Some children may have received their CIs before the presence of additional developmental disabilities (i.e., beyond hearing loss) could be detected . Thus, toddlers who have shown very limited changes in auditory and speech skills after one year of implant experience should receive a comprehensive interdisciplinary evaluation. The evaluation team typically includes parents, the child's EI, members of the implant team, a psychologist, a social worker, and personnel with expertise in any area of suspected disability. Broad-based assessment tools such as *Transdisciplinary Playbased Assessment* (Linder 1993) and the *Communication and Symbolic Behaviors Scales* (Weatherby and Prizant 1993) can be particularly useful in estimating the child's level of development because they assess a variety of communicative behaviors and are completed in naturalistic contexts. Evaluation results should lead to intervention strategies that meet the newly identified needs of the child while continuing to optimize opportunities for auditory learning.

Summary

Early intervention can lead to substantial improvements in listening, speech, and oral language for infants and toddlers who use CIs. This progress is facilitated as parents and interventionists work together to apply special techniques during daily interactions. Such collaborative efforts continue to be essential as children enter preschool. In addition, as children mature, clinician-directed intervention becomes an increasingly viable means of facilitating communication growth. The application of these instructional approaches with preschool children will be considered in Chapter 7.

Suggested Reading

▶ *Cochlear Implants for Kids*
Estabrooks, W. (1998)
Washington, D.C.: A.G. Bell Association

▶ *Baby Talk: Helping your Hearing-Impaired Baby Listen and Talk*
Kozak, V. J. and Brooks, B. (2001)
St. Louis: Central Institute for the Deaf

▶ *Listening for the Littles*
Sindrey, D. (1997)
London, Ontario: WordPlay Publishers

Internet Resources

▶ www.jamesmacdonald.org
Communicating Partners is a Web site devoted to parents who are helping their children develop social and communication skills.

▶ www.vocaldevelopment.com
An interactive Web site that contains audio recordings of various types of vocalizations, video examples of speech and language stimulation techniques, and information about early speech development.

▶ www.jtc.org
The Internet site of the John Tracy Clinic contains information about correspondence courses for parents of children who are deaf or hard of hearing.

▶ http://www.learningtolisten.org/pavt.html
The Web site for the Learning to Listen Foundation offers parent support, lesson plans, and answers to frequently asked questions about Auditory-Verbal therapy.

References

Bernthal, J. E. and Bankson, N. W. (1988). *Articulation and phonological disorders* (2nd Ed). Englewood Cliffs, NJ: Prentice Hall.

Brackett, D. and Zara, C. (1988). Communication outcomes related to early implantation. *American Journal of Otology*, 19, 453-460.

Brown, R. (1973). *A first language: The early stages.* Cambridge, MA: Harvard University Press.

Donahue-Kilburg, G. (1992). *Family-centered early intervention for communication disorders: Prevention and treatment.* Gaithersburg, MD: Aspen Publishers, Inc.

Ertmer, D. J. and Galster, J. (2001). *Vocal development.com.*

Ertmer, D. J. and Mellon, J. A. (2001). Beginning to talk at 20 months: Early vocal development in a young cochlear implant recipient. *Journal of Speech-Language and Hearing Research*, 44, 192-206.

Ertmer, D. J. and Stark, R. E. (1995). Eliciting prespeech vocalizations in a young child with profound hearing impairment: Usefulness of real-time spectrographic displays. *American Journal of Speech-Language Pathology*, 4, 33-38.

Ertmer, D. J., Young, N., Grohne, K., Mellon, J. A., Johnson, C., Corbett, K., et al. (2002). Vocal development in young children with cochlear implants: Profiles and implications for intervention. *Language, Speech, and Hearing Services in Schools*, 184-195.

Estabrooks, W. (1998). *Cochlear implants for kids.* Washington, D.C.: A.G. Bell Association.

Fenson, L., Dale, P., Resnick, J., and Bates, E. (1993). *MacArthur communication development inventories: User's guide and manual.* San Diego: Singular.

Kent, R. D., Osberger, M. J., Netsell, R., and Hustedde, C. G. (1987). Phonetic development in identical twins differing in auditory function. *Journal of Speech and Hearing Disorders*, 52, 64-75.

Kuhl, P. K. and Meltzoff, A. N. (1996). Infant vocalizations in response to speech: Vocal imitation and developmental change. *Journal of the Acoustical Society of America*, 100, 2425-2438.

References, *continued*

Leonard, J. S. (1992). Communication intervention for children at risk for specific communication disorders. *Seminars in Speech and Language*, 13, 223-235.

Linder, T. W. (1993). *Transdisciplinary play-based assessment*. Baltimore: Paul H. Brookes.

Ling, D. and Ling, A. H. (1978). *The foundations of verbal learning in hearing-impaired children*. Washington, D.C.: A.G. Bell Association.

McCaffrey, H. A., Davis, B. L., MacNeilage, P. F., and von Hapsburg, D. (1999). Multi-channel cochlear implantation and the organization of early speech. *Volta Review*, 101, 5-28.

Moeller, M. P. (2000). Intervention and language development in children who are deaf and hard of hearing. *Pediatrics*, 106(3), E43.

Nathani, S., Ertmer, D. J., and Stark, R. E. (2002). *The Stark assessment of early vocal development-revised*. Paper presented at the annual convention of the American Speech-Language and Hearing Association, Atlanta, GA.

Oller, D. K. (1980). The emergence of the sounds of speech in infancy. In G. Yeni-Komshian, J. Kavanaugh, and C. Ferguson (Eds.), *Child phonology* (pp. 93-112). New York: Academic Press.

Oller, D. K. (2000). *The emergence of the speech capacity*. Mahwah, NJ: Lawrence Erlbaum Associates.

Oller, D. K. and Eilers, R. (1988). The role of audition in infant babbling. *Child Development*, 59, 441-449.

Robbins, A. (2003). Communication intervention for infants and toddlers with cochlear implants. *Topics in Language Disorders*, 23, 16-33.

Robbins, A. M. and Kirk, K. I. (1996). Speech perception assessment and performance in pediatric cochlear implant users. *Seminars in Hearing*, 17, 353-369.

Robbins, A. M., Koch, D. B., Osberger, M. J., Zimmerman-Phillips, S., and Kishon-Rabin, L. (2003, April). *Effect of age at implantation on auditory skill development in infants and toddlers*. Paper presented at the Ninth Symposium on Cochlear Implants in Children, Washington, D.C.

Rossetti, L. M. (2001). *Communication intervention: Birth to three*. San Diego, CA: Singular-Thompson Learning.

The Source for Children with Cochlear Implants　　　　96

References, *continued*

Stark, R. E. (1980). Stages of speech development in the first year of life. In G. Yeni-Komshian, J. Kavanaugh, & C. Ferguson (Eds.), *Child phonology* (Vol. 1, pp. 73-90). New York: Academic Press.

Stark, R. E. (1983). Phonatory development in young normally hearing and hearing-impaired children. In I. Hochberg, H. Levitt, & M. J. Osberger (Eds.), *Speech of the hearing-impaired: Research, training, and personnel preparation*. Baltimore: University Park.

Stoel-Gammon, C. and Otomo, K. (1986). Babbling development of hearing-impaired and normally hearing subjects. *Journal of Speech & Hearing Disorders*, 51, 33-41.

Templin, M. (1957). *Certain language skills in children*. Minneapolis, MN: University of Minnesota Press.

Vihman, M. M. (1996). *Phonological development: The origins of language in the child*. Cambridge, MA: Blackwell.

Vihman, V. M., Ferguson, C. A., and Elbert, M. (1986). Phonological development from babbling to speech: Common tendencies and individual differences. *Applied Psycholinguistics*, 7, 3-40.

Wetherby, A. and Prizant, B. (1993). *Communication and symbolic behaviors scales*. Chicago, IL: Riverside Publishing.

Yoshinaga-Itano, C. (2000). Development of audition and speech: Implications for early intervention with infants who are deaf or hard of hearing. *Volta Review*, 100, 213-236.

Yoshinaga-Itano, C., Sedey, A. L., Coulter, D. K., and Mehl, A. L. (1998). Language of early- and later-identified children with hearing loss. *Pediatrics*, 102(5), 1161-1171.

Zimmerman-Phillips, S., Osberger, M. J., and Robbins, A. (1997). *Infant-toddler meaningful auditory-information scale*. Sylmar, CA: Advanced Bionics Corporation.

Communication Intervention for Preschoolers with Cochlear Implants

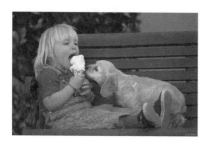

The preschool years provide a wealth of occasions for social and communicative growth in children with cochlear implants (CIs). Playing with friends, interacting with teachers, listening to stories, participating in preschool routines, and learning pre-academic skills afford many opportunities for improving listening, speech, and language skills. Yet, factors such as age-at-implantation, length of implant experience, amount of pre-implant hearing, family involvement, and communication modality can influence how well children take advantage of these situations. Whether attending a regular preschool or one for children with hearing loss, it is essential that parents, teachers, and clinicians, coordinate their efforts to help young CI users take full advantage of their improved hearing ability. This chapter will examine the roles of each of these stakeholders, and present assessment procedures and intervention approaches for meeting the communicative needs of preschool children who use CIs.

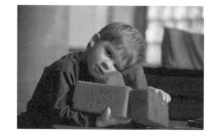

Parents, Teachers, and Clinicians Working Together

Involving Parents

Communication intervention during the preschool years focuses on two main goals: stimulating the development of auditory, speech, and language skills and helping children become successful communicators in everyday situations. As with infants and toddlers, parents continue to be unique and valuable resources for addressing these goals.

Parental perceptions of their child's strengths and needs can provide key information for developing effective Individualized Educational Plans (IEPs). For instance, parents can often identify specific communication needs that would make a big difference in the child's life. These can be as basic as helping the child recognize and say a classmate's name or as advanced as reinforcing irregular past tense verbs in spontaneous speech. Parents also know a great deal about how to motivate their children. Knowledge of the child's interests can help the clinician design engaging intervention sessions that have greater potential for generalization to everyday situations.

Parents also play an indispensable role in oral language development by continuing to use the interaction enhancement techniques and communication strategies described in Chapter 6. Language facilitation takes on added importance as children attempt to acquire the vocabulary and language skills needed to "keep up" with classmates. Thus, active parent involvement remains a vitally important part of communication intervention at the preschool level.

Wilkins and Ertmer (2002) have highlighted a number of ways that parents can become actively involved in their child's preschool. In addition to regular conferences with teachers and clinicians, passing a notebook between home and school on a daily basis can ensure that parents are aware of preschool news; current listening, speech, and language goals; and other classroom-related topics. Parents can, in turn, use the notebook to let school personnel know how the child is progressing at home, to share interesting family events, to ask questions, and to make comments and suggestions.

Counseling Teachers

Clinicians who work in regular preschools also need to help classroom teachers understand the special needs and abilities of children with CIs. This counseling should include discussions of the types and causes of hearing loss, the impact of hearing loss on language development, and strategies for optimizing communication and learning in the classroom. Resources for these discussions can be found in the books and Web sites listed on pages 124 and 125 respectively. It is also essential that teachers have a basic understanding of how a cochlear implant works, how to do daily listening and troubleshooting checks, and the need to avoid sources of electro-static discharge (e.g., plastic playground equipment). This information can be found in the implant owner's manual or in brochures prepared especially for teachers. The latter can be ordered on-line at implant manufacturers' Web sites. Other school personnel (i.e., principal, bus driver, teacher aides) should also be familiarized with the implant and its care so that problems outside of the classroom can be avoided.

The interaction enhancement and language facilitation techniques described in Chapter 6 should also be shared with the classroom teacher and teacher aides. Aside from parents, these professionals have the greatest number of opportunities to support the child's oral language development. Helping them understand why and how language facilitation techniques should be used will increase opportunities for communication development throughout the day. As previously discussed, it may be most helpful to demonstrate— rather than describe—a few input, response, and clarification strategies, and to encourage teachers to use the techniques that they find most comfortable.

Combining Clinician-Directed Instruction and Language Facilitation Techniques

Because of their increased maturity, many preschool children with CIs are able to benefit from clinician-directed instruction (Fey 1986), as well as from the continued use of language facilitation techniques previously described in Chapter 6. Using these approaches concurrently enables clinicians to stimulate the development of basic speech perception and speech production skills through guided practice, while also promoting language acquisition in the context of naturally occurring interactions.

Clinician-directed intervention involves the use of structured situations in which listening, speech production, or language targets are introduced and practiced in a concentrated way. Key elements of clinician-directed instruction include repeated modeling and elicitation of target behaviors; the use of auditory, visual, and tactile cues; reinforcement of correct responses; feedback on correctness; an emphasis on self-evaluation; and generalization of learning to more complex and less-structured contexts.

Although CIs increase the potential for incidental language learning, the continued presence of hearing difficulties (e.g., poorer than normal aided hearing sensitivity levels and trouble understanding speech in noise) can interfere with the efficient development of speech perception and production skills. The combination of clinician-directed instruction and language facilitation techniques can help overcome these problems and maximize auditory-oral learning potential. Basic procedures for two clinician-directed activities, auditory training and speech production training, are presented next.

Auditory Training

Auditory training has been defined as "instruction designed to maximize an individual's use of residual hearing by means of both formal and informal listening practice" (Tye-Murray 1998, p. 503). There are three commonly used approaches to auditory training: analytic, synthetic, and pragmatic. Taken together, these approaches are intended to improve children's ability to detect, discriminate, identify, and comprehend spoken language in a variety of situations. Analytic and synthetic auditory training will be discussed in this chapter because they are crucial for developing basic speech perception skills and communication abilities. Pragmatic auditory training focuses on preventing and overcoming communication breakdowns. These tasks require a level of metacognitive ability and assertiveness that is usually beyond preschoolers, and so they will be considered in Chapter 8.

Analytic Auditory Training

(Adapted from Ertmer 2002 with permission from the American Speech-Language-Hearing Association)

Children with CIs are faced with the challenge of becoming auditory-oral communicators after a period of auditory deprivation. How well this challenge is met depends, to a great extent, on how well they learn to detect and discriminate differences between speech sounds. Analytic auditory training is a "bottom-up" approach that seeks to enhance auditory skills by contrasting the "parts of speech" (i.e., suprasegmental characteristics and vowel and consonant features) so that a full range of speech sounds can be recognized (Blamey and Alcantara 1994). When using an analytic approach, grossly different sounds are contrasted first, and increasingly finer acoustic distinctions are introduced later.

Research has shown that suprasegmental patterns (e.g., stress and timing) and vowel features are easier for children with CIs to identify than consonant manner, voicing, and place cues (Fryhauf-Bertschy et al. 1997, Miyamoto et al. 1992). These findings provide the basis for the curriculum described in *Contrasts for Auditory and Speech Training* (*CAST*) (Ertmer 2003), an analytic auditory training program for children with cochlear implants. Table 7.1 on pages 102 and 103 lists the seven levels included in the *CAST* curriculum, the suprasegmental and segmental contrasts covered, and the numbers of the picture cards representing each contrast. Analytic auditory training activities are usually conducted in a quiet setting so that target speech features are not masked by environmental noises.

In analytic auditory training, minimal pairs are used to present examples of speech sound contrasts. For example, the minimal pair words *fan* and *tan* can be used to contrast fricative and stop consonants, respectively. Speechreading cues are also minimized so that children learn to recognize speech features through audition alone. This is accomplished by using an acoustic screen (an embroidery hoop covered with two layers of loosely woven cloth; see Figure 5.1, page 65) to cover the speaker's mouth as stimulus items are presented. Although *CAST* procedures will be used to illustrate analytic auditory training in this chapter, similar procedures are also used in auditory training programs such as the *Speech Perception Instructional Curriculum and Evaluation* (Moog et al. 1995) *and CHATS*: *The Miami Cochlear Implant, Auditory and Tactile Aid Curriculum* (Vergara and Miskiel 1994).

Table 7.1: CAST Levels of Analytic Auditory Training
Pretest (cards 1-28) (dark blue*)

I. Identification of suprasegmental cues (red*)

- Presence vs. Absence of Speech (cards 29-34)
- Long vs. Short Productions (cards 35-40)
- Continuous vs. Interrupted Sounds (cards 41-46)
- Words differing by syllable number
  - ▸ 1- vs. 3-Syllable Words (cards 47-60)
  - ▸ 1- vs. 2-Syllable Words (cards 61-74)
  - ▸ 2- vs. 3-Syllable Words (cards 75-88)

II. Identification of phonemically dissimilar words (green*)

- 1-Syllable Words (cards 89-102)
- 2-Syllable Words (cards 103-110)

III. Minimal pair words for vowel contrasts (yellow*)

- Wide Vowel Contrasts (cards 111-122)
  - ▸ i, ɑ, u, o, æ
- Narrow Vowel Contrasts
  - ▸ i/ɪ (cards 123-126)
  - ▸ ɛ/ɪ (cards 127-130)
  - ▸ ɛ/æ (cards 131-134)
  - ▸ ɑ/o (cards 135-138)
  - ▸ ɑ/æ (cards 139-142)
  - ▸ u/o (cards 143-146)

IV. Minimal pair words for consonant manner contrasts (orange*)

- Stops/Fricatives (cards 147-152)
- Stops/Affricates (cards 153-158)
- Stops/Liquids (cards 159-164)
- Stops/Glides (cards 165-170)
- Stops/Nasals (cards 171-176)
- Nasals/Fricatives (cards 177-182)
- Nasals/Affricates (cards 183-188)
- Nasals/Liquids (cards 189-194)
- Nasals/Glides (cards 195-200)
- Fricatives/Liquids (cards 201-206)
- Fricatives/Glides (cards 207-212)

Table 7.1: CAST Levels of Analytic Auditory Training, *continued*
• Fricatives/Affricates (cards 213-218) • Affricates/Glides (cards 219-224) • Liquids/Affricates (cards 225-230)
V. Minimal pair words for consonant voicing contrasts (purple*)
• f/v (cards 231-234) • s/z (cards 235-238) • p/b (cards 239-242) • t/d (cards 243-248) • k/g (cards 249-252) • dʒ/tʃ (cards 253-256)
VI. Minimal pair words for consonant place contrasts (pink*)
• p/t/k (cards 257-264) • f/s/ʃ (cards 265-272) • l/r (cards 273-276) • m/n (cards 277-280) • b/g/d (cards 281-286)
VII. Minimal pairs differing in final consonants (cards 287-300) (cyan blue*)
* The *CAST* cards are color-coded by section. This color indicates the bar color for this section. (Ertmer, D., *Contrasts for Auditory and Speech Training*, 2003)

Many three- and four-year-olds can successfully participate in analytic auditory training if activities are relatively brief and presented in a game-like way. Pairing stimulus sounds with toy figures (e.g., a prolonged "baaaaa" with a sheep vs. a short "tweet" with a bird) and using reinforcers (e.g., puzzle pieces or tokens) can make training seem more like play. There are eight basic steps for auditory training using the *CAST* materials.

1. *Select a starting point.* Begin at *CAST* Level I if the child is newly implanted. For children with more CI experience, use the *CAST* pretest to determine which contrasts are identified with less than 75% accuracy and begin training at that level.

2. *Introduce the contrast items.* Once a beginning level has been chosen, select a contrast for auditory training. These can be nonwords (e.g., continuous vs. interrupted sounds: /a/ vs. /a/ /a/ /a/) or words (e.g., *pop* vs. *mop*). To introduce the selected contrast, say each word/non-word stimulus item several times as you point to the picture or object that it represents. For example, if contrasting one- vs. three-syllable words, say "car" and "Popsicle" several times in random order as you point to the corresponding pictures. Asking personally meaningful questions about the items (e.g., "What color is your car?" or "What kind of Popsicle do you like?") can help the child remember the items. Provide more spoken models and identification practice if the child seems unsure of the association between the stimulus items and their associated pictures/objects. Ask the child to point and label each picture before going to step three.

3. *Present one of the stimulus items.* Using an acoustic screen to cover your mouth, say one of the stimulus items at a slightly louder than conversational level.

4. *Have the child respond.* The child should repeat the same stimulus item aloud and then point to the corresponding picture/object.

5. *Reinforce correct responses.* Give positive feedback when the child identifies items correctly. Although the child may mispronounce the item, keep the primary emphasis on auditory rather than speech production skills.

6. *Deal with errors.* There are three main options for responding to errors. They should be selected according to the needs and learning style of the child.

   a) Indicate that a mistake has been made, repeat the item, and ask the child to respond again. Although this option is sometimes effective, it also makes it very easy for the child to identify the correct answer by guessing.

   b) Ignore mistakes and provide feedback only when the child is correct. This option assumes that the child will learn to identify the contrast with continued exposure and positive feedback.

   c) Use a combination of auditory and visual cues:

      1) Get the child's attention and then cover your mouth with the acoustic screen as you say the item again.

      2) Put the screen down and let the child see your mouth as you say the word once more.

      3) Cover your mouth with the screen as you say the word a third time. Ask the child to say and point to the picture before presenting additional stimuli in random order. This option is intended to help the child associate speech reading cues with auditory cues, and should be faded to encourage auditory-only recognition (Koch 1999).

7. *Keep things moving.* Present ten words/non-words in random order for each selected pair of contrasts. Stimulus items should be presented at a brisk pace so that the activity is completed in a relatively short amount of time (e.g., five to seven minutes). For preschool children, one to two sets of contrasts can be presented per session. Older children may be able to complete more sets in a comparable amount of time. Analytic listening practice should be kept short to maintain children's attention and to allow time for other speech production and language activities within the same session.

8. *Record performance data.* Document percent correct scores for each session. It is suggested that new minimal pairs and contrasts from higher levels be introduced when the child is ≥80% accurate for two consecutive sessions.

The following modifications can be used to make analytic auditory training more engaging and effective. They can be applied to school-age as well as preschool children.

Modifications for Analytical Auditory Training Activities
(Adapted from Ertmer et al. 2002, Robbins 1990, Tye-Murray 1993)

1. Whenever possible, incorporate personally meaningful words in training. For example, family member names, spelling words, numbers, words from finger-plays, and reading vocabulary words, increase the likelihood of improved listening in everyday situations. Gather objects, draw pictures, take photographs, or write words on blank cards to represent these new items. Personally meaningful words are especially important during the early stages of auditory training and should be reinforced at home and in the classroom.

2. Young children may maintain interest better when each response is rewarded with a game or puzzle piece. For example, the child may be given a marble for every correct response. These can be dropped in a marble maze when a certain number of marbles have been earned.

3. Include progressively longer and more difficult materials (e.g., three or more choices, longer carrier phrases and sentences, multiple step directions) as the child's listening abilities improve. For example, four pictures can be placed on the table for practice in following three-part directions (e.g., "Touch *gate* and *kite* before *light*") or negatives ("Point to *dock* and *yak* but not *lock* or *tack*").

4. Keep listening activities light by the use of positive feedback, encouragement, false assertions, and humor. Unexpected but familiar words (e.g., the child's name, favorite food) can be interspersed with target contrasts during training activities. Inserting unexpected words makes listening practice more unpredictable and helps to keep the child alert for irregularities in everyday communication (e.g., *kite, bite, Batman*).

5. Frequently allow the child to assume the role of the "talker" as you take the role of the listener. This "turnabout" helps to enhance speech production as well as speech recognition skills.

6. Include a variety of male and female talkers in auditory training whenever possible. Include children as well as adults.

7. Include contrasts in the final and medial, as well as initial positions in words.

Finally, it is important to remember that some older children, especially those with late onset of deafness or those with several years of implant experience, may recognize speech features and identify minimal pair words with high accuracy. Speech perception tests may reveal that these children require little, if any, analytic training.

Synthetic Auditory Training

Children with CIs are asked to comprehend conversations with family, friends, and teachers on a daily basis. Their success in these interactions can have a strong influence on their attitudes toward oral communication and their progress in developing speech perception skills. Synthetic auditory training is a top-down approach that places emphasis on comprehending spoken messages rather than recognizing the parts of the speech signal (Blamey and Alcantara 1994). Using this approach, phrases, sentences, and paragraphs are presented and children are asked to repeat them, answer questions, or demonstrate comprehension by participating in conversations. Synthetic auditory training is designed to help children learn to use available contextual, syntactic, and semantic cues to decipher the meaning of the messages they receive throughout the day. The following are examples of synthetic listening activities for preschool and school-age children.

1. Play "I See It" when looking at a picture book with large-scale scenes. For example, when looking at the beach scene in the *First 1000 Words* (Cartwright 2003), the clinician can say, "I see a boy with a blue swimsuit." The child listens and finds the boy before taking a turn at telling the teacher to find the next object or person. Theme-based picture books are also useful for introducing vocabulary words.

2. Use predictable books to highlight repeated phrases. For example, take turns identifying the blue horse, white dog, or goldfish from among other pictures in *Brown Bear, Brown Bear* (Martin 1995). See the Web site at the end of the chapter for a compilation of predictable books.

3. Play "Mother May I" by taking turns giving directions that should only be carried out if they include "Mother says…" and the child's response includes "Mother may I?" For example, the clinician says, "Mother says take two steps backward." The child says, "Mother may I?" The clinician answers, "Yes, you may." Take turns giving and following directions with groups of children.

4. Play "Treasure Hunt" by hiding written directions around the room. For example, the first note might say "Look behind the door." The second note could instruct the child "Open the door and turn right." Following these spoken directions eventually leads the child to the treasure.

5. Play barrier games in which both parties have the same sets of pictures/blocks/toys but cannot see the other's materials because of a barrier between them. The clinician and the child take turns telling the other how to arrange their materials, and then check to see how well the directions were followed.

6. Play the "Guess Who" game (Milton-Bradley) to see who can identify a person based on physical appearances.

7. Ask the child to construct objects using paper shapes. For example, make a sheep by using a large oval for the body, a circle for the head, and narrow rectangles for the legs. See how many other animals or objects can be made using the same set of colored shapes. Take turns giving directions.

8. Speech tracking (DeFillpo and Scott 1978) can be used with older elementary school children. "Tracking" activities require listeners to repeat sentences verbatim as stories, magazine articles, or newspaper items are read aloud to them. Repair strategies are used to help the listener when a message is not fully understood. For example, feedback on correctly identified words can be given, or the first sound in misunderstood words can be provided as a clue. Special care must be taken to match the language level of the reading materials to the child's abilities. Selected readings should also be related to the child's interests or school assignments.

The benefits of synthetic training are more likely to be generalized when the stimulus materials are relevant and interesting to the child. For example, young children are usually motivated to learn through theme-based activities that focus on family members, pets, games, foods, cartoons, toys, and stories. For older children, topics of personal interest (e.g., music, hobbies, movies, sports) and school-related concepts can enhance social and academic, as well as, listening skills. Additional ideas for preschool children can be found in *Listening for the Littles* (Sindrey 1997) and *Cochlear Implants for Kids*

(Estabrooks 1998). Activities and lesson plans for integrating listening and academics for school-age children can be found in the *Guide for Optimizing Auditory Learning Skills* (*GOALS*) program (Firszt and Reeder 1996).

Synthetic listening activities can also be integrated with language goals. For example, sentences with simple syntax (e.g., "I want X," "Give me Y," or "Where is Z?") can be used repeatedly with children who are just beginning to understand and use word combinations. Using typical patterns of language development as a guide, stimuli should be adjusted to include longer, more complex, and varied sentences as the child's language skills increase. Allowing children to take turns as talkers during listening/ language activities ensures that both auditory comprehension and verbal expression are emphasized.

In a very real sense, every conversation with the child is a synthetic auditory training experience. Thus, training can be conducted in both the auditory-only and the auditory-plus speechreading conditions, depending on the child's abilities and the clinician's instructional philosophy. The effectiveness of synthetic auditory training is evaluated as clinicians, parents, and teachers document improvements in understanding spoken language and participating in conversations.

Speech Development

Cochlear implants provide two main benefits for speech development in young children. First, improved access to conversational-intensity speech models and auditory feedback increases opportunities to develop speech through incidental learning. Secondly, CIs increase hearing sensitivity across the low, mid, and high frequency ranges. Having access to a wide range of spectral information supports the development of a complete inventory of speech sounds.

Although improved hearing sensitivity can lead to more normal patterns of speech development, there are two compelling reasons to expect that young children with CIs will require assistance to develop speech efficiently. First, it must be remembered that implanted children have had a late start in auditory-guided speech development. They are already significantly behind their age peers in speaking ability. Overcoming this deficit is likely to require special efforts to accelerate speech learning and to unlearn any previously adopted maladaptive speech production strategies (e.g., ingressive production of consonants, unusual substitutions; Higgins et al. 1996). Additionally, the aided thresholds of CI users do not usually fall within normal limits. Since speech production difficulties are often associated with mild and moderate levels of hearing loss, it seems reasonable to expect that children with CIs will also have problems in this area. The next section will discuss the kinds of assessments needed to develop speech intervention programs for children with CIs.

Speech Assessment

Six areas should be considered when assessing speech development in children with CIs. Information from each of these areas is essential for determining current speech production abilities, selecting intervention priorities, choosing intervention strategies, and estimating progress over time.

Assessment Areas and Tools

1. *Hearing sensitivity and auditory skills.* Effective speech intervention programs require a clear understanding of each child's auditory capabilities. Unaided and aided (with CI turned on) hearing sensitivity levels can be found in the child's audiologic folder. Aided thresholds can provide an estimate of the audibility of various consonants and vowels when plotted onto an audiogram that illustrates the intensity and spectral characteristics of speech sounds (see Figure 7.2 on page 112). Speech perception test results are used to estimate word and sentence recognition and comprehension abilities (see Chapter 2, page 28, for specific tests).

2. *Intraoral examination.* The structure and function of the oral mechanism are assessed through visual inspection of the lips, teeth, tongue, hard and soft palates, and pharyngeal area, and through elicitation of articulator movements. The purpose of this assessment is to identify abnormalities that may impact speech production. Results of this exam are shared with medical professionals if inadequacies are observed. See Paul (2002) for more information.

3. *Suprasegmental and phonation abilities.* The basic purpose of this assessment is to see how well children can control voicing. Imitative vowel productions are elicited to determine whether vocalizations can be initiated on demand, whether the duration of vocalizations can be varied, whether vocal intensity can be varied along a soft-loud continuum, and whether a range of pitches from low to high can be produced (Ling 1976, 1989). Voice quality and resonance are also observed during these tasks. Adequate phonatory control and acceptable voice quality should be considered intervention priorities if problems are noted.

Assessment Areas and Tools, *continued*

---

4. *Phonetic abilities.* Evaluation at the phonetic level involves having the child attempt to imitate a variety of speech segments in simple, non-meaningful contexts. For example, the Ling Phonetic Level Evaluation (Ling 1976, 1978) requires children to imitate vowels, diphthongs, and consonants in CV syllables. Phonetic evaluations are especially useful for children who do not say words on a regular basis.

5. *Phonologic abilities.* Children's ability to produce meaningful speech can be examined by administering articulation tests, analyzing speech samples, and completing the Ling Phonologic Level Evaluation (Ling 1976). The results of these assessments can be used to compare the child's level of speech development to that of normally hearing peers, to identify articulation errors and phonological processes, and to select targets for intervention. Follow-up stimulability testing should be used to determine whether error phonemes can be produced correctly after cues and/or facilitation techniques are provided. Phonemes that are stimulable for correct production may be acquired without speech training (Miccio et al. 1999).

6. *Speech intelligibility.* Speech intelligibility can be measured at the single word or sentence level by having judges listen to recordings of speech samples and make subjective ratings (e.g., good, fair, poor; five-point rating scale) or write down the words that are understood. The latter method yields a percent-intelligible word score. For authentic results, judges should not be familiar with the child's speech. Speech intelligibility scores should be gathered at least annually so that functional speech gains can be examined. See Osberger et al. (1993) for lists of short sentences appropriate for preschoolers and school-age children. *The Picture Speech Intelligibility Evaluation* (*Picture SPINE*) (Monsen et al. 1988) can be used to evaluate word-level intelligibility in school-age children.

Table 7.2: Audiogram for Estimating the Audibility of Voicing Cues and Phonemes Produced at Conversational Intensity Levels

Name: _____   Date: _____

Type of Cochlear Implant: _____   Processing Strategy: _____

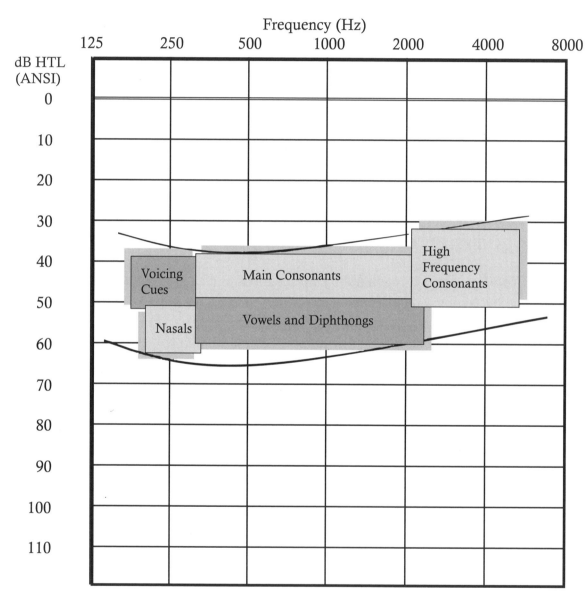

(Adapted from Risberg and Martony 1970)

Speech Facilitation

There are two main goals for phonological intervention with CI users between three and five years old:

- to help children learn how to produce a full range of vowels, diphthongs, and consonants correctly
- to facilitate the use of these speech sounds in meaningful speech

The title of this section is "speech facilitation" rather than "speech training" to emphasize the fact that—barring technical or learning problems—many young CI recipients can make substantial speech gains through exposure to conversational speech and auditory feedback. The aim of intervention then, is to support and accelerate this learning; rather than to correct misarticulated phonemes. To this end, speech facilitation consists of clinician-directed activities to expand phonological inventories and promote generalization of improved speech to everyday situations.

As described earlier in this chapter, children are asked to say a variety of speech sounds during analytic auditory training activities. Although this form of speech practice is very important for associating phonemes with the articulator movements that produced them, a more concentrated approach is needed to overcome speech delays. The intent of speech facilitation is to expose preschoolers to a wide range of phonemes, give opportunities to say these sounds in syllables and words, provide instruction to help children say targets correctly, and foster use of speech targets in spontaneous speech.

Decisions, Decisions

There are several fundamental decisions to make when planning speech facilitation for preschoolers. These include:

1. deciding how to engage young children in speech activities
2. selecting the order in which speech targets are presented
3. determining when to introduce new targets

Encouraging Active Participation. Engaging preschoolers in structured speech tasks can be tricky. Many can attend to direct instruction for short periods of time only. Thus, efforts to introduce and practice speech sounds must occur in the context of play-like activities. Here are some suggestions for making speech facilitation an enjoyable learning experience.

Young children may find it difficult to recognize and remember a variety of speech sounds. Associating them with metaphors for animal sounds (e.g., /r/ for tiger's growl), actions (e.g., blowing for /w/), or verbal expressions (e.g., [m:m:] for tasty food) can help them to recall and conceptualize phonemes more easily (see Bliele 1995 for a listing of metaphors).

Clinicians can also provide numerous models of speech targets through auditory bombardment or focused stimulation while the child is engaged in play. Such concentrated modeling is intended to increase awareness of speech targets across a variety of words. Auditory modeling periods should be followed by game-like activities that emphasize production of the same phonemes so that perception and production practice are closely coordinated (see Hodson and Paden 1991 for suggested activities).

Carryover can be encouraged through simple performances that include many opportunities to say targeted sounds. Children enjoy learning and performing finger-plays, poems, riddles, and songs. Arts and crafts activities, role-playing, and short "speeches" about a topic of interest (e.g., careers, families, pets, sports) can also be useful in transferring new sounds to spontaneous speech. See the Web sites on page 124 for language play activities that can be used to reinforce targets in connected speech.

Ordering Speech Targets. Clinicians have two main choices for selecting the order in which targets are presented. These include a developmental approach in which phonemes are introduced in the order they are mastered by children with normal hearing (e.g., Sander 1972, Selby et al. 2000), and the Ling Phonetic Level Curriculum (1976, 1989), in which speech goals have been designed especially for children with hearing losses.

Following a normal developmental sequence has several limitations for children with CIs. To begin with, stop and nasal consonants are emphasized during the early stages of intervention. However, children with CIs may make more rapid gains if a wider variety of sounds (including those with low-mid and high-frequency characteristics) are emphasized from the start. Secondly, following a developmental sequence does not address any basic phonatory or suprasegmental control problems that the child may have. For example, some children may need to master the basic skill of turning their voices on and off before focusing on expanding their consonant inventories. Finally, targeting single sounds in developmental order may not be time-efficient. That is, an approach in which sets of diverse sounds are introduced and practiced together can make speech feature contrasts more apparent. In summary, although following a normal developmental sequence appears to have face-validity, it does not provide an adequate range of auditory stimulation, address basic speech production issues, or facilitate the recognition of a wide range of speech sound contrasts. A more specialized approach is needed if speech learning is to be accelerated.

Although designed for children who use hearing aids, the Ling Phonetic Level Curriculum (1976) is well-suited to the speech needs of young cochlear implant users. This comprehensive program emphasizes the development of basic phonation skills, presents a hierarchy for expanding segmental inventories that is based on increasing reliance on audition, and employs speech sound contrasts to help children learn a variety of voicing, manner, and place distinctions. By including later-developing consonants (e.g., fricatives) across all steps, it also provides high frequency stimulation for the auditory nerve. Administering the Ling Phonetic Level Evaluation (1978) enables clinicians to determine an appropriate starting point for each child. In short, Ling's carefully constructed curriculum can help clinicians order the introduction of speech targets to maximize speech learning with a CI. Table 7.3 on page 116 presents sets of vowel, diphthong, and consonant sounds that can be introduced and contrasted/practiced together. Note that some sets contain cognates (i.e., consonants differing only in voicing). In these cases, one member of each cognate pair is introduced initially and the remaining one targeted later. Speech sounds that the child already says do not have to be practiced.

How Much Is Enough? The Ling approach provides a framework for introducing speech targets, but clinicians must decide how much attention each group of sounds should receive. This decision is based on children's proficiency in identifying and saying targets, by the amount of time available (i.e., if attempting to allocate similar amounts of time for each set of sounds), by children's interest levels, or by a combination of these factors. Children need not be highly accurate in producing each target before new sets of targets are introduced. Sounds that are slow to develop at first may become more acceptable through continued CI use. They can also be revisited later if production difficulties persist.

Table 7.3: Proposed Sequence for Speech Facilitation with Preschool Children (Adapted from Ling 1976)	
1. Vowels and Diphthongs Sets 1 – 4	/a, i, u, au, aɪ/ /ɔ, ɔɪ, ɛ, ʊ, ɪ/ /æ/, /ʌ/ or /ɑ/, /o/ /ɝ, ə, ɚ/
2. Simple Consonants Sets 1 – 3	/b/ or /p/ and /w/ or /ʍ/ /f/ or /v/ and /θ/ or /ð/ /h/ and /m/
Sets 4 – 6	/d/ or /t/ and /ʃ/ or /ʒ/ /s/ or /z/ and /n/ /l/ and /j/
Sets 7 – 8	/g/ or /k/ and /tʃ/ or /dʒ/ /ŋ/ and /r/
3. Consonant Blends One-organ blends Two-organ blends Single-organ conformulated blends Complex blends	/sm, sl, sn, st, θr/ /bl, br, fl, fr, kw, pl, pr, tw/ /dr, gl, gr, kr, ʃr, tr/ /skr, skw, spr, str/

Optimizing Speech Learning

The following suggestions are intended to help children make full use of their hearing capabilities and become actively involved in speech learning. They can be used with school-age as well as preschool children.

1. *Maximize the child's reliance on audition.* Introduce new sounds in the auditory-only condition by using an acoustic screen. Ask children to imitate what they hear. Visual and tactile cues can be provided if the child experiences extended difficulty in producing targets but should be faded as soon as possible.

2. *Trade roles with the child.* Let the child be the "teacher" while you model both correct and incorrect productions of the target. Ask the child to tell you how to improve your production.

3. *Encourage self-evaluation.* Once the child begins to modify his productions, shift the emphasis from clinician-provided feedback to child judgments. Use neutral terms (e.g., "Was that the old way or the new way to say X?") rather than "good" and "bad" to evaluate productions.

4. *Use encouragement more often than praise when giving feedback.* Encouragement highlights what the child has done right. For example, "I heard you say /f/" or "Your tongue stayed behind your teeth that time." In contrast, praise does not reinforce the desired speech behaviors directly and may not motivate some children.

5. *Have high expectations for speech sound carryover, but focus on the child as a communication partner first.* That is, listen to what the child is saying to you and respond accordingly. Try to make speech corrections meaning-based. For example, "You want my ba? Oh, you want my ball," rather than "Say ball again and remember the /l/ this time."

6. *Provide opportunities to "show off" newly-mastered sounds for parents, peers, and teachers.* Practice and perform poems, finger-plays, riddles, jokes, and plays that contain targets the child can say well. Keep in mind that some children may not enjoy performing for others. These children may be more comfortable demonstrating their abilities in conversational contexts.

7. *Keep parents and teachers informed of current speech targets.* Let them know when the child has made improvements. Encourage them to reinforce improved skills at home and in school.

Language Development

Language Assessment Tools for Children with CIs

As with children who have normal hearing, language assessments for preschoolers with CIs take three main forms: informal measures, criterion-referenced procedures, and norm referenced tests. *Informal measures* include observations of communicative behaviors (e.g., comprehension and use of words and sentences, communicative intents) in a variety of situations, interviews of parents and teachers, checklists of communication skills, and language samples. Many of the commercially available informal assessment tools developed for children with normal hearing can be used with young CI users. Clinicians will also find the *Spontaneous Language Analysis Procedure* (*SLAP*) (Kretschmer and Kretschmer 1978) helpful for language sample analysis because it was developed for children with hearing loss. *SLAP* examines both receptive and expressive language across a wide range of abilities. Informal measures are especially useful for assessing pragmatic language abilities and selecting functional communication goals.

Criterion-referenced procedures allow clinicians to measure how well a child can perform specific speech, language, or listening tasks. For example, a child may be asked to combine color and object names (e.g., white car) when presented with ten pictures. The child's score can serve as a baseline of ability and improvement can be estimated when the task is repeated at a later time. Criterion-referenced tasks can be easily constructed to measure specific language goals for individual children and are especially useful for documenting progress on IEPs.

The vast majority of commercially available *language tests* have been standardized on children with normal hearing. The reader is likely to be familiar with many of these and so they will not be reviewed here. Although these tests can be administered to CI users, it is important to interpret test results cautiously. If age and standard scores are calculated, it should be clearly indicated that they were derived from scores of children with normal hearing. Progress can be estimated by re-administering standardized tests at allowable intervals (e.g., six months or one year).

Several tests have been standardized on children with hearing loss. *The Grammatical Analysis of Elicited Language* (*GAEL*) (Moog and Geers 1985) has two forms: the Simple Sentence level and the Complex Sentence level. The first form measures comprehension and expression of single-word vocabulary and word combinations, and is often used with preschoolers. The Complex Sentence level examines the same domains for longer sentences and a variety of morphological markers. *The Test of Syntactic Abilities* (Quigley et al. 1978) and the *Rhode Island Test of Language Structure* (Engen and Engen 1983) also assess syntactic and morphologic knowledge. It should be kept in mind that norms for children with hearing loss are based on the performance of hearing aid users, and not children with CIs.

As with children who have normal hearing, a combination of informal, criterion-referenced, and norm-referenced measures is needed for a comprehensive picture of language ability.

The listening, speech, and language skills acquired during the preschool period serve as a base for social and academic growth in the elementary, middle, and high school years. Chapter 8 focuses on ways to further close the communication gap between children with CIs and their normally hearing peers.

Language Facilitation in Natural Contexts

Typically developing children acquire spoken language skills in the course of their everyday experiences. Because of their improved hearing abilities, such routine experiences have the potential to boost language development in young CI users as well. Although language deficits in older children are often addressed through clinician-directed activities, intervention for preschool children may be more effective when language facilitation techniques are employed in the context of naturally occurring conversations.

Judith Johnston (1984) has proposed several guiding principles for intervention with preschool children who have language disorders. These principles are based on presumed language acquisition processes in which learning is driven by the children's social needs, fueled by their cognitive resources, and guided by a search for ways to express ideas. Accordingly, the purpose of intervention is to accelerate the course of language development while maintaining the essence of these natural language learning processes. To this end, Johnston proposes the guiding principles of *Fit*, *Focus*, and *Functionality* as means to tailor language intervention to the individual preschool child. Although originally proposed for normally hearing children who have language disorders, these principles appear to be well-suited for children with CIs who experience language learning delays due to prelingual deafness and residual hearing problems.

Increasing Fit, Focus, and Functionality. *Fit* involves matching language content (i.e., linguistic targets/models/input) and instruction to the individual child's abilities and learning styles. Fit is achieved when selected language targets build on children's established language behaviors, and intervention strategies take into account the child's nonverbal knowledge and range of communicative intents. *Focus* involves helping children learn language rules by narrowing and simplifying their search for linguistic regularities. Focus is achieved when language models are modified to highlight linguistic rules and targets while restating the child's intended message. *Functionality* means targeting language constructions that children will use in everyday interactions. Functionality is achieved when selected language targets have direct relevance to the child's everyday communication needs. Table 7.4 on pages 121 and 122 contains suggestions for individualizing language facilitation during child-initiated activities.

Table 7.4: Suggestions for Increasing Fit, Focus, and Functionality of Language Intervention (Adapted from Johnston 1984)	
Improving Fit	**Match input to the child's developmental level.** 1) Use normal patterns of language development as a guide (e.g., Brown 1973). 2) Select language targets that are slightly more advanced than the child's current level. **Match input to the child's learning style.** Give input using the verbal and non-verbal communication intents (e.g., commenting, requesting, negation) that the child already uses. **Match input to the way the child uses language.** 1) Does the child use language primarily to describe or refer to objects, or does the child use language primarily for self-expression and social interactions? Model in a similar way. 2) Does the child appear to learn single words and then combine them to make longer phrases, or does the child appear to produce longer utterances and then "break-down" the components? Model in a similar way. 3) Children focus on meaning more than language structure. Describing easily interpretable events (e.g., the "here and now") simplifies understanding and allows the child to pay more attention to the "fading acoustic event" that is speech (Johnston 1984, p. 130).
Increasing Focus	**Modify your models to highlight selected linguistic targets.** Use these techniques as you provide models or restate the child's intended messages. 1) Present consecutive examples of the target. 2) Present the target multiple times. 3) Present the target at the end of a phrase/sentence. 4) Stress the target by making it slightly louder and/or longer. 5) Use melodic intonation to call attention to the target. 6) Provide new vocabulary for any indefinite words. 7) Associate words and referents (e.g., "The boy has a car. **He** has a car"). Use targets in contexts where meaning is easily understood, such as during play and daily routines.

Table 7.4: Suggestions for Increasing Fit, Focus, and Functionality of Language Intervention, *continued*	
Achieving Functionality	**Use input to help the child communicate.** 1) Provide words and constructions that the child can use in the current situation. 2) Provide words and constructions that the child needs for other play and social situations. 3) Develop play activities that require the child to use language to get what is desired. For example, put a favorite snack in a difficult to open container so that the child must request help. 4) Take advantage of naturally occurring situations for language facilitation throughout the day. For example, introduce new vocabulary and language structures when the child notices unfamiliar items, events, or situations.

Verbal Reasoning and Literacy

It is important to remember that, in addition to interpersonal communication, language is also a tool for reasoning and for acquiring knowledge. Parents, teachers, and clinicians can foster the development of verbal reasoning by sharing their thought processes aloud. Taking the time to predict daily events out loud (e.g., "I think Daddy's knocking at the door"), explaining the causes of puzzling events (e.g., "He's crying because he has a headache"), reading books daily, discussing the calendar and scheduled events, naming objects in the child's environment, and discussing natural occurrences (e.g., "We have to wear coats today. It's almost winter") can help children to understand their world and to make inferences. Establishing and following daily routines can also give children a sense of the future and the past. Verbal reasoning skills should be emphasized from a young age so that a solid foundation is laid for social and academic success.

Exposure to printed language can also open doors to a wider world. Pre-literacy activities such as tracing and naming letters, posting printed labels on household objects, and "reading" business signs and logos around the community alert children to the communicative power of printed symbols. Children's literature can be especially useful in helping young CI users make sense of what they hear. By listening to the same story several times, children begin to understand that sounds and written symbols are related, that different readers are saying the same words (even though they don't sound exactly the same), and that they can say the same words to "read" the story themselves.

Two forms of children's literature are especially valuable for developing language and literacy skills in preschool children. As the name implies, ***wordless picture books*** portray a story without printed words. The pictures convey all of the meaning. Because there are no printed words to follow, adult readers can easily match their narratives to the child's language level from single words to complex sentences. Wordless books also encourage children to retell the story using their own words. Verbal reasoning is enhanced as the children interpret the pictures, make inferences about story events, and come to realize that stories have a beginning, a middle, and an end. A Web site for wordless picture books can be found on page 124.

Predictable books are also quite useful for preschoolers and elementary children. These appealing stories have some repeated or predictable patterns that entice children to make guesses about words, phrases, or outcomes. After listening to a predictable story once, children often want to hear it again so they can say the pattern on their own. Repeated readings may lead to children insisting on "reading" the entire story without help. A Web site for predictable books can be found on page 124.

Suggested Reading

▶ *Facilitating Hearing and Listening in Young Children*
Flexer, C. (1999)
San Diego: Singular

▶ *Understanding Hearing Loss*
Lysons, K. (1996)
London: Jessica Kingsley Publishers

▶ *Preschool Language Disorders Resource Guide*
Weiss, A. L. (2001)
San Diego: Singular

▶ *Speech Disorders Resource Guide for Preschool Children*
Williams, A. L. (2003)
Delmar Learning: Clifton Park, NY

Internet Resources

▶ http://www.agbell.org
Information and resources on hearing loss, sensory aids, classroom issues. Brochures and related books can also be ordered.

▶ http://education.qld.gov.au/curriculum/learning/students/disabilities/index.html
Information regarding hearing losses of varying degrees and inclusive education for children with impaired hearing.

▶ http://www.listen-up.org
Information across a wide range of hearing-related topics. Links to hearing loss simulations and many other useful sites.

▶ http://www.preschoolrainbow.org/preschool-rhymes.htm
A resource for preschool activities, themes, and creative ideas for young children.

▶ http://www.zelo.com/family/nursery/
An alphabetical listing of nursery rhymes for preschoolers.

▶ http://www.monroe.lib.in.us/childrens/predict.html
A catalog of predictable books for young children.

▶ http://www.weberpl.lib.ut.us/child_wordless.htm
A compilation of wordless picture books.

References

Blamey, P. J. and Alcantara, J. I. (1994). Research in auditory training. *Journal of the Academy of Rehabilitative Audiology*, 27 (Suppl.), 161-192.

Bliele, K. M. (1995). *Manual of articulation and phonological disorders: Infancy through adulthood.* Clifton Park, NY: Delmar Learning.

Brown, R. (1973) *A first language: The early stages.* Cambridge, MA: Harvard University Press.

Cartwright, S. (2003). *First thousand words.* London: Usborne Publishers.

DeFillippo, C. and Scott, B. (1978). A method for training and evaluating the reception of ongoing speech. *Journal of the Acoustical Society of America*, 63, 1189-1192.

Engen, E. and Engen, T. (1983). *Rhode Island test of language structure.* Baltimore: University Park Press.

Ertmer, D. J. (2002). Auditory training for school-age children with cochlear implants: Addressing speech perception and oral communication needs. *Perspectives on Hearing and Hearing Disorders in Childhood*, 12, 29-32.

Ertmer, D. J. (2003). *Contrasts for auditory and speech training (CAST).* East Moline, IL: LinguiSystems, Inc.

Ertmer, D. J., Leonard, J. S., and Pachuilo, M. L. (2002). Communication intervention for children with cochlear implants: Two case studies. *Language, Speech, and Hearing Services in Schools,* 33(3), 205-217.

Estabrooks, W. (1998). *Cochlear implants for kids.* Washington, D.C.: A.G. Bell Association.

Fey, M. (1986). *Language intervention with young children.* Needham Heights, MA: Allyn & Bacon.

Firszt, J. B. and Reeder, R. M. (1996). *GOALS: Guide for optimizing auditory learning skills.* Washington, D.C.: A.G. Bell Association.

Fryhauf-Bertschy, H., Tyler, R., Kelsay, D., Gantz, B., and Woodworth, G. (1997). Cochlear implant use by prelingually deafened children: The influence of age at implant and length of device use. *Journal of Speech, Language & Hearing Research*, 40, 183-199.

References, *continued*

Higgins, M. B., Carney, A. E., McCleary, E., and Rogers, S. (1996). Negative intraoral air pressures of deaf children with cochlear implants. *Journal of Speech and Hearing Research*, 39, 957-967.

Hodson, B. and Paden, E. (1991). *Targeting intelligible speech: A phonological approach to remediation.* Austin, TX: Pro-Ed.

Johnston, J. R. (1984). Fit, focus, and functionality: An essay on early language intervention. *Child Language Teaching and Therapy*, 1, 125-134.

Koch, M. (1999). *Bringing sound to life.* Baltimore: York Publishing.

Kretschmer, R. and Kretschmer, L. (1978). *Language development and intervention with the hearing impaired.* Baltimore, MD: University Park Press.

Ling, D. (1976). *Speech and the hearing-impaired child: Theory and practice.* Washington, D.C: A.G. Bell Association.

Ling, D. (1978). *Teacher/Clinician planbook and guide to the development of speech skills.* Washington, D.C.: A.G. Bell Association.

Ling, D. (1989). *Foundations of spoken language development.* Washington, D.C.: A.G. Bell Association.

Martin, B. (1995). *Brown bear, brown bear, what do you see?* New York: Holt & Company.

Miccio, A., Elbert, M., and Forrest, K. (1999). The relationship between stimulability and phonological acquisition in children with normally developing and disordered phonologies. *American Journal of Speech-Language Pathology*, 8, 347-363.

Miyamoto, R. T., Osberger, M. J., Robbins, A. M., Myres, W. A., Kessler, K., and Pope, M. L. (1992). Longitudinal evaluation of communication skills of children with single- or multi-channel cochlear implants. *American Journal of Otology*, 13(3), 215-222.

Monsen, R. B., Moog, J., and Geers, A. (1988). *Picture speech intelligibility evaluation.* St. Louis: Central Institute for the Deaf.

Moog, J. and Geers, A. (1985). *Grammatical analysis of elicited language.* St. Louis: Central Institute for the Deaf.

References, *continued*

Moog, J. S., Biedenstein, J. J., and Davidson, L. S. (1995). *Speech perception instructional curriculum and evaluation.* St. Louis: Central Institute for the Deaf.

Osberger, M. J., Maso, M., and Sam, L. K. (1993). Speech intelligibility of children with cochlear implants, tactile aids, or hearing aids. *Journal of Speech and Hearing Research,* 36, 186-203.

Paul, R. (2002). *Introduction to clinical methods in communication disorders.* Baltimore, MD: Brookes Publishing Company.

Quigley, S. P., Steinkamp, M., Power, D., and Jones, B. (1978). *The test of syntactic abilities.* Beaverton, OR: Dormac.

Risberg, A. and Martony, J. (1970). A method for the classification of audiograms. In G. Fant (Ed.), *Speech communication and profound deafness* (pp. 135-139). Washington, D.C.: A.G. Bell Association.

Robbins, A. M. (1990). Developing meaningful auditory integration in children with cochlear implants. *Volta Review,* 96, 361-370.

Sander, E. (1972). When are speech sounds learned? *Journal of Speech and Hearing Disorders,* 37, 55-63.

Selby, J. C., Robb, M. P., and Gilbert, H. R. (2000). Normal vowel articulation between 15 and 36 months of age. *Clinical Linguistics & Phonetics,* 14, 255-266.

Sindrey, D. (1997). *Listening for the littles.* London, Ontario: WordPlay Publishers.

Tye-Murray, N. (1993). Aural rehabilitation and patient management. In R. S. Tyler (Ed.), *Cochlear implants: Audiological foundations* (pp. 87-144). San Diego: Singular Publishing Group.

Tye-Murray, N. (1998). *Foundations of aural rehabilitation.* San Diego: Singular Publishing Group.

Vergara, K. C. and Miskiel, L. W. (1994). *CHATS: The Miami cochlear implant and tactile aid curriculum.* Miami, FL: Intelligent Hearing Systems.

Wilkins, M. and Ertmer, D. J. (2002). Introducing young children who are deaf or hard of hearing to spoken language: Child's Voice, an oral school. *Language, Speech, and Hearing Services in Schools,* 33, 196-204.

Communication Intervention for School-Age Children with Cochlear Implants

8

If you are a school-based speech-language pathologist, an educational audiologist who provides aural habilitation in the schools, or a teacher of the hearing-impaired, the chances of having a child with a cochlear implant (CI) on your caseload are steadily increasing. To date, more than 10,000 children have received cochlear implants in the United States. Many of these were implanted as infants or toddlers and were eventually enrolled in preschool programs that emphasize the development of oral communication skills. Graduates of these programs are often integrated into regular kindergarten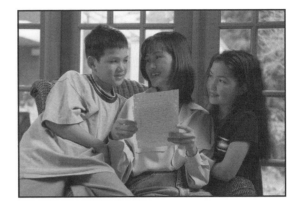
or first grade classrooms in neighborhood schools. Other children have received their implants while enrolled in special classrooms or schools for children with hearing loss. Many of these children eventually enter regular classrooms as well. In fact, a recent study has shown that 75% of children from a large metropolitan area were enrolled in regular classrooms within four years of receiving their implants (Niparko et al. 2000). More children with CIs than ever before are receiving communication intervention in regular schools.

School-age children with cochlear implants show considerable heterogeneity in their listening, speech, and language skills. As a result, clinicians are challenged to develop highly individualized intervention plans. This chapter offers several frameworks to help meet this challenge. The reader should keep in mind, however, that there are few, if any, studies of intervention effectiveness for this population. Thus, the ideas proposed in this chapter are based on previously developed models, related research, and practitioner experience, rather than the results of treatment efficacy studies.

Children with CIs must be able to communicate effectively in a number of settings and situations: at home, in school, with peers, and with adults. Achieving this ambitious goal requires the coordinated support of many individuals. This chapter will begin with a discussion of the roles of school professionals, parents, and the implant team, and the benefits of establishing a collaborative working relationship among these stakeholders.

Working with Parents, Teachers, and the Implant Team

Although intervention strategies change as children with CIs grow-up, collaboration among concerned stakeholders remains vitally important throughout the school years. The human pyramid (Figure 8.1) is used to symbolize how parents, teachers, clinicians, extended family, and friends provide a base of support for helping children with CIs to develop their talents. In addition to supporting children as they acquire communication, social, and academic skills, stakeholders support each other in many ways. This support includes sharing information about the child's progress, recognizing the importance of each stakeholder's efforts, and reinforcing each other's goals for the child.

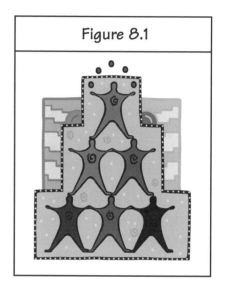

Figure 8.1

Parents as Resources

Parents of children with CIs can be a well-spring of information and insights for school-based professionals. Of all parties, they have the greatest knowledge of their child's abilities and needs. This knowledge was gained as they participated in the implant evaluation; monitored their child for gains in listening, speech, and language skills; and dealt with implant technology and its inherent problems. In short, parents can be remarkable resources for setting goals, developing instructional strategies, and for stimulating and reinforcing learning. Clinicians and teachers can tap into these resources by actively listening to parents' concerns and ideas, and by exchanging information frequently throughout the school year.

Opportunities to develop a mutual support system arise as parents and professionals meet to share information, review multi-disciplinary testing results, and develop an Individualized Educational Plan (IEP) during the initial school-based case conference. This conference is usually scheduled before the child begins to attend regular classes. The main purposes of the meeting are to identify any special educational, physical, and social needs that the child may have; formally enroll the child in appropriate remedial/support services; develop an IEP; and specify the amount of special assistance needed. Special classroom modifications and instructional accommodations may also be considered at this time (see Chapter 9).

It is especially important that school personnel understand the abilities and needs of children with cochlear implants. Many classroom teachers are unfamiliar with basic information regarding the effects of hearing loss on oral communication, CI technology, and procedures and safeguards for implant use. Much of this information can be found in the Resources and Web site sections of Chapter 7, in Chapter 1, and in the CI owner's manual, respectively. Special booklets for teachers are also available from implant manufacturers. Sharing technical information with teacher aides and other school personnel (i.e., the principal, bus drivers, and playground supervisors) can help to ensure the safety of the child and the proper care of the implant in all settings.

Collaborating with Teachers

Clinicians and classroom teachers must work closely together if children's communication and academic progress are to be maximized. Clinicians will need the teacher's help to identify children's communication strengths and needs, and to reinforce newly learned language, speech, and communication skills. In return, they should identify ways to incorporate classroom curriculum into intervention sessions as much as possible. Suggestions for addressing communication and literacy in an integrated way will be offered later in this chapter. Good communication between parents, classroom teachers, special educators, and communication specialists can help to optimize social and academic success. Frequent conferences, phone calls at regular intervals, and use of a home-school notebook ensure that stakeholders support each other as well as the child.

Communicating with the CI Team

In addition to working closely with parents and teachers, school clinicians will want to communicate regularly with the CI team. Written reports from the implant center provide the most reliable estimates of the child's hearing sensitivity and speech perception ability, as well as suggestions for maximizing auditory learning. This information is essential for designing intervention programs. Copies of these reports can be obtained by having the parents fill out a Health Insurance Portability and Accountability Act (HIPAA 1996) "Release of Information" form at the implant center. This document specifies the information that you are requesting (i.e., audiograms, test scores, and reports related to auditory-oral functioning) and the purpose for requesting the information (i.e., for intervention planning). Parents may also choose to share their copies of the child's evaluation reports with you. School-based clinicians should contact the parents if the child's speech and listening abilities appear to worsen. For example, a consistent decrease in the ability to imitate Ling sounds (see page 30) or declines in vowel and consonant accuracy during spontaneous speech may indicate that the implant map or the implant itself has been damaged. Similarly, reduced ability to identify words and sentences during auditory training and conversation can be a sign of technical problems. If routine maintenance (e.g., replacing a cord or installing fresh batteries) does not fix the problem, parents will need to schedule an appointment at the implant center and to make arrangements for a "loaner" speech processor until the child's unit can be repaired.

Representatives of the implant team should be invited to special educational conferences whenever the child is experiencing difficulty in developing auditory-oral, social, or academic skills. Clinicians should also feel free to consult with members of the implant team who specialize in communication intervention. These professionals have many resources for enhancing auditory-oral communication.

Speech Perception and Auditory Comprehension

Assessment

The characteristics of speech perception tests have been reviewed on page 28 of Chapter 2. School-based communication specialists need to be familiar with this information because implant centers routinely use speech perception tests to assess post-implantation progress. Speech perception testing is usually conducted by implant audiologists under very controlled conditions (i.e., presentation of prerecorded stimulus materials at a selected intensity level in a sound booth) so that reliable estimates of improvement can be made over time. Although center-based assessments are essential for monitoring CI benefit, testing within the school setting can also yield useful information for intervention planning.

Several speech perception tests can be used to select "starting points" for analytic auditory training (see Chapter 7, page 101). These can be administered face-to-face in a quiet room if clinicians present the stimuli at close-to-conversational intensity level while using an acoustic screen (page 65). Examples of these tests include the

Cottage Acquisition Scales for Listening, Language, and Speech (Wilkes 1999), the *Early Speech Perception Test for Profoundly Hearing-Impaired Children* (Moog & Geers 1990), and the *Contrasts for Auditory and Speech Training Pretest* (*CAST*; Ertmer 2003). Each of these instruments provides an indication of the child's ability to recognize words and non-words through listening alone. Because they are based on a hierarchy of auditory skills, auditory training usually begins at the point where a child first experiences difficulty recognizing speech contrasts.

Several tests that have been developed for children with normal hearing are helpful for estimating auditory comprehension ability and for planning synthetic auditory training activities (see Chapter 7, page 108). For example, the *Revised Token Test For Children* (RTTFC, DiSimoni 1978) examines a child's ability to understand increasingly complex spoken directions when vocabulary is limited to a small set of sizes, shapes, colors, and prepositions. If the vocabulary is familiar to the child, *RTTFC* results can give an estimate of the length of utterance that the child comprehends. *The Listening Test* (Barrett et al. 1992) examines the ability to understand main ideas, remember details, understand concepts, use reasoning, and comprehend stories through listening. Although this test does not control for vocabulary or sentence length, the tasks are comparable to those found in many classroom situations. Gains in auditory comprehension can be estimated by re-administering these tests annually. It is also important to remember that assessments of auditory comprehension should also include conversational samples and parents' and teachers' observations of the child's ability to understand spoken language at home and school.

Pragmatic Auditory Training

Children with cochlear implants can "miss out" on large amounts of auditory information during their everyday interactions with teachers, friends, and parents. To make matters worse, they often pretend to understand when they do not. This section describes pragmatic auditory training, an approach for avoiding and dealing with communication breakdowns.

Communication breakdowns often occur when the spoken message is masked by environmental noises, as the distance between the talker and the listener increases, when excessive reverberation causes distortion of the message, and when the language of the message is not understood. Pragmatic auditory training provides children with facilitative and repair strategies to improve communication in such difficult listening situations.

Facilitative communication strategies include statements and requests that influence the talker to speak more slowly, provide better speechreading cues, or simplify the message. They also include actions to optimize listening in difficult environments and attempts to anticipate the content of conversations. For facilitative strategies to be effective, children must anticipate or recognize the sources of listening difficulty and respond to them in an assertive way. Table 8.1 contains examples of difficult listening situations and potential facilitative strategies. Clinicians are encouraged to help the child develop personalized and preferred expressions/responses to these situations so that they are more likely to be remembered and used.

Table 8.1: Examples of Difficult Listening Situations and Facilitative Communication Strategies		
	Situations	Examples of Strategies
Strategies to Influence the Talker	The talker is facing away from me when speaking.	I will move so I can see the talker's face better.
	The talker speaks too quietly/ too softly.	"I can't understand you. Please speak a little slower/louder."
Strategies for Influencing the Message	The message is complex or lengthy.	"What do you mean?" Can you say that another way?"
	The vocabulary is unfamiliar.	"I don't know what 'foul ball' means."
Strategies that Influence the Environment	The hallway is too noisy.	I will ask to have my desk moved away from the hall door.
	I can't hear the whistle during gym class and miss part of what the teacher says.	I will ask the gym teacher to get my attention before she starts to give directions.
Strategies that Influence the Way the Listener Receives a Message	Sometimes my attention drifts when people talk to me.	I'll try to look at the talker's mouth and rephrase what she says from time to time.
	I am meeting people for the first time and want to be sure I can carry on a conversation.	I'll ask mutual friends about their interests so I can talk about them. I'll be prepared to introduce a familiar topic, if necessary.

Whereas facilitative strategies can help to avoid communication breakdowns and influence future interactions with the same talker, ***communication repair strategies*** are used immediately after a breakdown occurs. Table 8.2 provides a listing of expressions that call for the talker to clarify information. In general, polite requests are much more acceptable than saying "Huh?" in response to a misunderstanding. Revealing one's hearing loss and providing feedback on exactly what has been understood can also help to lessen the talker's frustration with being asked to repeat a message.

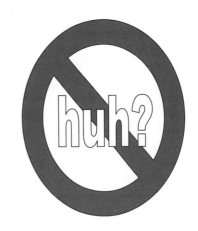

Table 8.2: Examples of Communication Repair Strategies
• Please say that again. I didn't hear you.
• I heard you say "Wednesday," but I missed the time we're going to meet.
• Could you ask me again? I had trouble understanding you with my cochlear implant.
• Did you say "stream" or "scream"?
• I heard you say something about soccer, but I missed the rest of it.

Although these strategies may appear to be common sense, they can be difficult to apply at first. Children typically require explicit instruction (e.g., modeling, practice with feedback, role-playing, clearly-stated expectations for use, and reinforcement) before they begin to understand when and how to use communication repair strategies. Clinicians, teachers, and parents should monitor and encourage the use of pragmatic strategies throughout the day so that bluffing is reduced. See the recommended reading list on page 159 for more information on pragmatic auditory training and communication strategies.

Three-in-One: An Eclectic Approach to Auditory Training

Children with CIs have both developmental and functional listening needs. That is, they must learn to recognize differences between speech sounds (a developmental need) and comprehend spoken messages throughout the day (a functional need).

Accordingly, auditory training must be broad-based enough to effectively address these needs. Programs that focus solely on analytic auditory training—a practice that Robbins (1994) has termed "greenhousing" because of its potential for limiting generalization of improvements—fail to address the child's functional, everyday communication needs. Similarly, those that focus solely on the comprehension of spoken messages do not directly deal with underlying deficits in the detection, discrimination, and identification of speech feature contrasts: foundational elements of spoken language. Additionally, intervention programs that ignore the consequences of difficult listening situations fail to help children overcome the communication breakdowns that they encounter frequently. An eclectic approach to auditory training addresses all of these needs by providing analytic, synthetic, and pragmatic training activities concurrently (Blamey and Alcantara 1994; Ertmer 2002).

Implementing an eclectic approach may seem unwieldy at first glance. After all, children with CIs are likely to have many speech and language goals, as well as the need for improved listening skills. How can all three of these areas be addressed in the limited time available? The answer to this question lies in session efficiency and integration of goals. Specifically, auditory discrimination and identification skills can be addressed efficiently by providing short periods of analytic training (approximately five minutes) during each session. A short time frame ensures that children have opportunities to become aware of speech sound distinctions without an overemphasis on de-contextualized listening practice. Synthetic auditory training—practice in comprehending spoken messages—can be easily integrated into activities that focus on speech and language development (more on this later in the chapter). Finally, although children often need direct instruction and practice with facilitative and communication repair strategies at first, once understood, they can be easily reinforced during the course of other activities. For example, children can be expected to say "I didn't understand you" or "Tell me again," as needed, while listening to stories in class or to instructions during intervention sessions. In short, although analytic auditory training requires short periods of decontextualized practice, efforts to increase comprehension of meaningful speech should be integrated with activities to improve the children's speech, language, and communication abilities.

Speech Production

Assessment

As mentioned at the start of the current chapter, school-age children with CIs will vary greatly in their speech production abilities. Newly implanted children may resemble younger children in terms of the relatively small number of speech sounds that they produce correctly. In contrast, children with many years of implant experience, strong speech perception ability, or a postlingual onset of hearing loss (among other possible influences) may have speech that is quite intelligible. The majority of school-age implant users will fall between these extremes, exhibiting various levels of speech proficiency and intelligibility. As with preschoolers, clinicians should examine speech production abilities by evaluating each of the six areas described in Chapter 7 on pages 110 and 111.

Observations of children's spontaneous speech can be used to select an appropriate speech production test. School-age children with very limited speech ability—those who say very little or produce few vowels or consonant types—will require a phonetic evaluation similar to the one proposed by Ling (1976, 1989; see Chapter 7, Assessment Areas and Tools, p. 111). Phonetic evaluations examine speech at a syllabic level, through imitation. In this way, language deficits do not interfere with speech testing. Children who consistently express themselves with spoken language can be evaluated at the phonological level through the production of words and sentences. Many commercially available articulation tests can be used to assess phonological development in children with CIs. It is important to remember, however, that children will differ in the degree of severity of their speech problems: some may have a few, unrelated misarticulations, while others may have sets of errors that reflect a common production constraint or phonological process. As is true for children with normal hearing, these two situations call for different intervention approaches (Bleile 1995). Although there are many useful speech assessment tools to choose from, two tests are particularly helpful in making this distinction.

The *Assessment Link between Phonology and Articulation-Revised* (*ALPHA-R*; Lowe 2000) and the *Goldman-Fristoe Test of Articulation-2* (Goldman and Fristoe 2000) in combination with the *Khan-Lewis Phonological Analysis-2* (Khan and Lewis 2002) allow the clinician to decide whether there is a need to analyze phonological processes as well as articulation errors. The *ALPHA-R* is especially valuable for children with CIs because it examines vowel as well as consonant production, a feature not found on many articulation tests. Similarly, the *GFTA-2* has the advantage of eliciting both words and connected speech through picture-naming and story-retelling tasks, respectively.

Clinicians will also want to consider the manner in which the words or sentences are elicited during testing. Children with limited vocabularies may be unable to name stimulus pictures spontaneously, and those with short MLUs may have trouble producing sentences. For such children, spoken models will be needed to elicit imitative responses. The use of models and imitation should be noted in evaluation reports so that results can be interpreted accordingly. As discussed in Chapter 7 (page 111), follow-up stimulability testing can be useful in prioritizing speech training goals.

Children's suprasegmental speech characteristics should also be examined. Spontaneous speech samples can reveal whether children typically speak at an appropriate intensity level, whether their rate of speaking is within normal limits (approximately four syllables per second; Lehiste 1970), and whether variations in intonation and stress are present and used appropriately. Step 1 of the Ling Phonetic Level Evaluation (Ling 1976, 1989) can be used to determine whether the child can alter pitch, intensity, and duration of speech sounds. Proficiency in using suprasegmentals in connected speech can also be assessed by having the child imitate sentences varying in loudness, stress placements, and intonation patterns. Speech that is overly slow, monotone, or that has little variation in stress can be hard to understand, and will call unwanted attention to the talker. Thus, goals for improving the use of suprasegmental features should be included in IEPs as needed.

Speech Production Intervention

School-age children with well-functioning CIs often make substantial improvements in speech skills through a combination of implant experience and clinician-directed intervention (e.g., Conner et al. 2000, Blamey et al. 2001). These gains are closely tied to their speech perception abilities. That is, children who have relatively greater speech production skills are also likely to be good perceivers of speech. Because of their increased auditory abilities, many of the conventional speech training methods used with children who have normal hearing are also appropriate for CI users. Rather than reviewing familiar articulation and phonological intervention techniques, the remainder of this section will offer suggestions to improve three areas of potential difficulty for children with CIs that are not common to children with normal hearing.

Vowel Production Errors

Vowel development is not usually a problem for children with normal hearing. Typically developing children learn to produce a full range of vowels by their third birthdays (Stoel-Gammon and Herrington 1990), and they learn to do so without any formal instruction. Vowel errors are also relatively scarce in children with normal hearing who have phonological delays or disorders. In contrast, the vowels of children with severe and profound hearing losses who use hearing aids are often inaccurate, limited in variety, and negatively impact speech intelligibility. Although children with CIs have been shown to increase their vowel inventories and production accuracy (Ertmer 2001, Tye-Murray and Kirk 1993), some school-age children may not produce a full range of vowels and diphthongs. In particular, front and back vowels can be relatively difficult for children with CIs (Tye-Murray and Kirk 1993).

One way to increase vowel production accuracy is to combine speech training with analytic auditory training. Using this approach, minimal pair words serve to increase awareness of the acoustic differences between vowel types while also providing multiple opportunities to produce vowel targets. For example, if a child substitutes /ɪ/ for /i/, he would listen as the clinician says stimulus words such as *bit* and *beat* or *fill* and *feel*, repeat the stimulus word after the clinician, and then point to the corresponding picture. This listen-say-point process integrates auditory and speech practice while encouraging self-evaluation. Reversing talker and listener roles can also motivate children to figure out how to produce vowel targets correctly, so that the clinician can identify the child's intended word. Generalization to more complex contexts can begin as acceptable vowels are produced consistently in contrasted words. See Chapter 7 for more information on analytic auditory training and suggestions for modifying minimal pair activities.

Atypical Suprasegmental Speech Patterns

A recent case study of a perilingually deafened CI user showed that children who acquire fairly good segmental speech skills may, nonetheless, have difficulties developing suprasegmental skills (Ertmer et al. 2002). "Drew" was a typically developing child prior to experiencing a bout with meningitis at three years. His resultant moderate hearing loss in the right ear and severe loss in the left ear remained relatively stable until he was seven years old. At that time his acuity levels suddenly decreased to the profound range of hearing loss in both ears. He received a CI shortly after becoming deaf. Drew made substantial gains in both speech perception and production during the first year of implantation. Although he mastered a variety of vowel, consonant, and consonant-blend targets, his spontaneous speech was atypically "soft" in intensity and lacking in intonation.

Several techniques were used to increase vocal intensity to more acceptable levels. First, Drew was asked to listen to the clinician as he spoke words at soft, medium, and loud levels, and then point to corresponding pictures of a child with a hand next to the mouth (quiet talking), a child with a slightly open mouth (normal talking), or a child with a wide open mouth (talking loudly), respectively (see Figure 8.2). Drew was then asked to "be the teacher" and say words and sentences at each intensity level while the clinician pointed to the corresponding pictures. These activities increased his awareness of and ability to produce speech at different intensity levels.

Drew was also asked to describe picture stories and converse loudly enough so that the clinician could hear him when sitting approximately ten feet away. This activity provided practice in sustaining comfortable, but adequately loud speech. Once aware of different loudness levels, Drew was encouraged to speak at an acceptable loudness level and monitor his intensity level throughout the day. Parents and teachers were also asked to reinforce appropriate vocal intensity at home and school.

Several techniques were used to increase intonation variation in spontaneous speech. At first, Drew was asked to listen to and sing familiar songs (e.g., "Happy Birthday," "The ABC Song"), and produce vowels with "pitches" that matched notes played on a small xylophone. These activities were intended to help him discover and produce a wider range of vocal tones. Next, Drew imitated sentences using different stress and intonation patterns (see Table 8.3 on page 142). Throughout these activities, intonation was associated with steady, rising, or falling pitch through line drawings: ——— , ———╱ , ———╲ , respectively. Stress was equated with increased loudness and/or increased duration. In addition to adding stress and intonation to these sentences, Drew was encouraged to figure out the meaning that was added by stressing a given word in the sentence (e.g., "I thought you went **home** after school, not somewhere else").

Figure 8.2: Drawings to Help Children Distinguish Between Quiet, Conversation-level, and Loud Speech

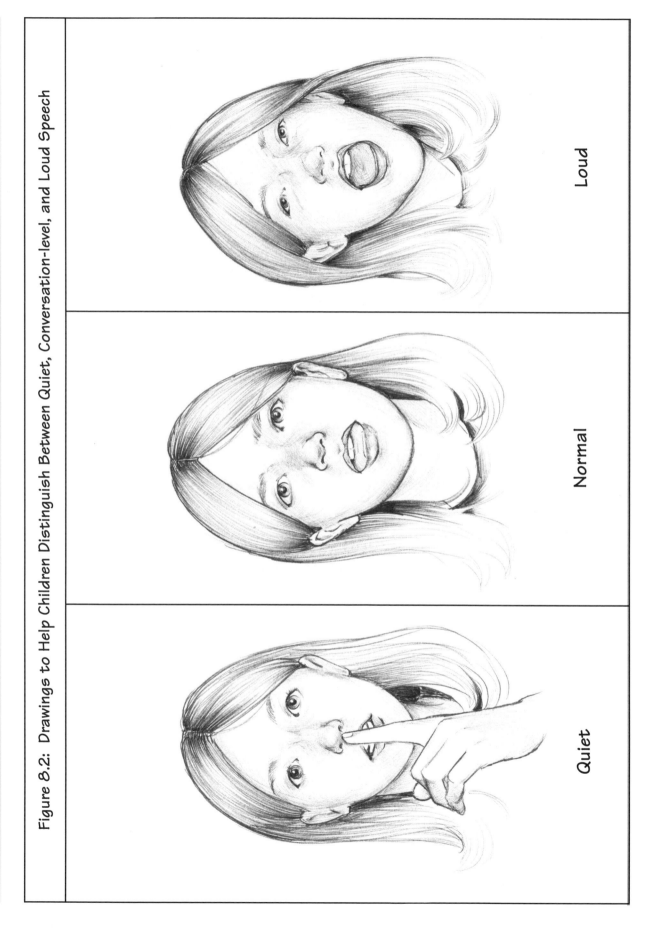

Quiet

Normal

Loud

Table 8.3: Examples of Sentences Used to Increase Use of Stress and Intonation Patterns
1. You went to the game last night.
2. You went to the game last night**?**
3. **You** went to the game last night?
4. You went to the **game** last night?
5. You went to the game **last night?**

Slow Speaking Rate

The speech of children with severe and profound hearing loss is typically quite slow. Despite their improved hearing, some children with CIs may need special practice to achieve an acceptable speaking rate. Ling (1976, 1989) addresses slow speaking rate by emphasizing the rapid production of syllables early in the speech training process. For example, children who are learning to produce /s/ are expected to say /s/-syllables at a rate of three per second or faster. Both repeated (e.g., sisisi) and alternated syllables (e.g., sasisasisasi, satasatasata) are practiced. Consonant targets are combined with a variety of front, central, and back vowels until a wide range of combinations can be produced rapidly. Vowel targets are alternated with different consonants using the same criterion. A near-normal rate of production is also emphasized for phrases and sentences.

Improvements in spontaneous speaking rate are likely to occur gradually as gains in segmental and suprasegmental abilities are made. Although a normal rate of speaking is desirable, readily intelligible speech remains the ultimate goal of intervention. To this end, some children may continue to talk at a slightly slower than normal rate in order to make themselves understood.

Language and Communication

Assessment

This section deals with the nuts and bolts of examining language and communication abilities in children with CIs. It includes discussions of three major types of assessments and suggestions to ensure that testing procedures help children perform to the best of their abilities. The reader is also referred to the language assessment section found in Chapter 7 for related information.

Testing Basics

Children with CIs require special consideration during language assessments. The following basic procedures can mean the difference between conducting a reliable testing session and gathering questionable results under frustrating conditions for the child.

1. Conduct testing in a room that is quiet, free from visual distractions, and has adequate lighting.

2. Sit across the table from the child so that speechreading cues are available for the child to use.

3. Check implant functioning by asking the child to imitate Ling sounds and by looking at the indicator lights on the speech processor. Ask the child if the CI is working properly before giving tests. Reschedule the session if there are technology problems.

4. Be sure that the evaluation is conducted using the child's mode of communication (e.g., Oral Simultaneous Communication or Cued Speech). An interpreter should be used if you are not a proficient signer. Be aware that some signs are iconic and may provide visual cues to the correct response.

5. Use a combination of formal tests, informal measures (e.g., language samples and criterion-referenced tasks), and observations of communication interactions to develop a comprehensive picture of the child's abilities and needs. These types of assessment are discussed next.

Types of Language and Communication Assessments

Formal Testing. As was true for speech tests, most standardized language tests have been developed for children with normal hearing. Many of these can be quite useful in estimating semantic, syntactic, and morphological abilities in children with CIs. A detailed discussion of these tools is beyond the scope of this chapter. Instead, clinicians are urged to keep three cautions in mind when using standardized tests with children who have CIs.

First, it is important to remember that *some test errors may be due to misperception of speech, rather than deficits in language skills or knowledge.* For example, if a child perceives "Dean" instead of the stimulus word "team," he may point to a picture of an individual rather than a group of children. Thus, clinicians should consider perceptual as well as linguistic reasons for the children's responses. For picture-identification tasks, auditory perceptual problems can be lessened by having the child repeat test items aloud before pointing to an answer.

It is also important to remember that *most language tests are decontextualized.* That is, the items have little or no relationship to each other. For example, syntactic ability might be assessed by asking children to imitate consecutive, unrelated sentences such as "My ball is red," "The large black dog is sleeping," and "The boy was chased by the girl." Children may perform poorly on such items because they lack the contextual cues found in conversations. Two exceptions to this situation can be found in the *Test of Semantic Skills—Primary* (*TOSS-P*) (Bowers et al. 2002) and the *Test of Semantic Skills—Intermediate* (*TOSS-I*) (Bowers et al. 2004). Both of these standardized tests incorporate stimuli from common childhood experiences (i.e., activities in a classroom, a store, or on a playground) with test items that are related to specific themes. Language samples also provide opportunities to examine the child's communication skills in context-rich situations and should be included in every evaluation.

Finally, *care should be taken not to overemphasize differences between the implant user's scores and those of children with normal hearing.* Children with CIs have less hearing experience than their age peers and should not be expected to match peer performance without extended use of their implants. Although raw scores, language ages, standard scores, and percentiles are sometimes required for enrollment in communication intervention programs, these scores have the most legitimacy when used to document within-child progress. In short, standardized test scores should be interpreted carefully and less-formal assessment procedures should be used to augment their findings. Two types of informal assessments will be discussed next.

Criterion-Referenced Testing. Criterion-referenced tasks consist of commercially available scales or clinician-constructed tasks that focus on specific language skills or knowledge (Miller and Paul 1995). For example, clinician-constructed tasks might require the child to use present progressive verbs to describe ten action pictures, or ask the child to follow 20 directions that contain prepositions. A set criterion (e.g., 80% correct) is used to determine whether intervention with the selected targets is warranted. Thus, criterion-referenced testing enables clinicians to determine the severity/consistency of problems, identify and prioritize treatment targets, and monitor progress by children with CIs.

Language Sampling. Formal language tests do not always reflect the child's true language abilities. Thus, it is recommended that such testing always be supplemented by language samples that include transcripts of both the child's remarks and those of a communication partner (Kretschmer and Kretschmer 1978). This type of sampling allows clinicians to identify language structures that are delayed in development and to determine how well children exchange ideas in meaningful situations. Having transcripts of both communicators provides the context necessary to understand the children's conversational abilities and needs. Such information is indispensable for developing an intervention program that addresses both children's language deficits and their functional communication needs.

Observations of Communication Interactions. In addition to standardized testing, criterion-referenced tasks, and language samples, it is essential to examine the child's communicative competence during a variety of social situations. Table 8.4 on page 146 contains a list of questions for assessing communicative behaviors at home and school. These questions should be jointly discussed by parents, teachers, and clinicians so that functional communication goals can be developed and supported by all stakeholders. A framework for improving communication ability through conversation-based intervention will be described in the next section of this chapter.

The Source for Children with Cochlear Implants   145

Table 8.4. Questions for Assessing Communicative Behaviors at School and Home

1. How often does the child respond to communicative attempts by others?

2. How often are the child's responses appropriate and related to the previous remarks of the communication partner?

3. How often does the child initiate communication? Is this a concern to parents and teachers?

4. What kinds of communicative intents does the child use appropriately (e.g., requesting, clarification, commenting, instruction giving, explaining, and persuasion)?

5. Can the child tell a story of more than three events? Are personal narratives easy to follow?

6. How does the child react to problems? Does he identify a range of possible solutions?

7. What factors interfere with communication among peers (e.g., speech intelligibility, failure to comprehend, lack of interest, shyness, physical aggression)? What communication goals does the classroom teacher have for the child?

8. How well does the child communicate at home? What concerns do the parents have? What communication goals do parents have for the child?

Language and Communication Intervention

Kretschmer (1997) and Wood and Wood (1997) have provided strong rationales for developing language and communication skills through conversations, rather than relying exclusively on traditional intervention methods (i.e., clinician-directed instruction). They note that children with normal hearing acquire language through conversations with adults and peers, that sharing (rather than controlling) a conversation causes adults to use more mature language models, and that participation in conversations allows children to utilize their cognitive abilities, to apply linguistic knowledge, and to connect new ideas with their own experiences (i.e., develop schemata [Yoshinaga-Itano and Downey 1986]).

As opposed to traditional intervention methods that emphasize mastery of language structures (e.g., comprehension and production of past tense verbs), communication-based intervention seeks to engage students in authentic conversations so that meaning can be constructed jointly, and relevant ideas, feelings, and reactions shared between adult and child (Kretschmer 1997). This approach is more than "just talking." For it to be effective, clinicians must be attentive to children's communicative and linguistic needs, address these needs through a variety of strategies (e.g., modeling, explaining, and connecting new information with the child's prior knowledge), and measure progress in terms of communicative improvements rather than mastery of language forms. Although clinicians may continue to use traditional instruction to introduce and practice some language structures, it is hoped that the following discussion will illustrate the potential advantages of a communication-based approach for developing functional communication skills, expanding vocabulary, increasing pragmatic skills, and integrating academic content into intervention activities.

Kretschmer proposes that school-age children with hearing loss must have adequate discourse skills with six communicative functions to be successful in social and academic situations. These functions include problem-solving, narration (i.e., storytelling), description, explanation, instruction-giving, and persuasion. Young, typically developing children acquire these communication skills primarily by interacting with parents and peers and by overhearing conversations. In contrast, children with CIs—because they begin to hear later in life and have relatively poorer access to ambient language models—are likely to need substantial conversational practice to develop age-appropriate use of communicative functions. Additionally, Greenberg (1993, cited in Kretschmer 1997) has noted that children with hearing loss are rarely exposed to the thought processes that adults use to solve problems. Thus, authentic conversations and "thinking aloud" are basic components of a communication-based intervention program.

Table 8.5 on pages 148-150 contains suggestions for enhancing the six communicative functions mentioned above. These activities should be considered as examples only. Conversational topics should be selected according to children's ages, abilities, and interests.

Table 8.5. Examples of Activities to Improve the Use of Communication Functions	
Communication Function	**Activities**
Problem-Solving	▶ The clinician describes a personal situation that needs to be resolved (e.g., knowing that you'll be late to pick up children at a game), discusses options that are available, and the pros and cons of each option. Ask the child to help you choose the best course of action to solve your problem. ▶ Clinician and child discuss a real-life classroom or playground problem, options, and select preferred actions to resolve it. Involve friends and the teacher if desired. ▶ Read an Aesop fable. The clinician takes the part of the main character and discusses the problem, options, and merits of various solutions. Ask the child to think up other choices. Reverse roles as you read another fable. ▶ Play "What would you do if..." Possible scenarios include: being locked out of your house, being lost downtown, and having a bad stomachache while on the bus. Take turns thinking through the options and deciding on a course of action. Discuss why various options would be acceptable/unacceptable.
Personal and Literary Narration	▶ The clinician shares a personal story (e.g., going on vacation or adopting a pet). Use chronological markers such as *first*, *second*, and *finally*. Ask the child to tell about a similar experience. Review the order of the events. ▶ Ask the child to tell a personal story as you chart the events by writing them down or drawing simple pictures. Have the child retell the story to parents and teachers while using the written text or illustrations. ▶ Have the child get ready to tell a personal story to a friend. Consider the information that the friend does/does not need to know (i.e., leave out the parts that the friend already knows about but include information that is new).

Table 8.5. Examples of Activities to Improve the Use of Communication Functions, *continued*	
Communication Function	**Activities**
Personal and Literary Narration, *continued*	▶ The clinician retells a familiar story while leaving out key elements (e.g., whose house Little Red Riding Hood visited). Ask the child to "remind" the clinician of the important parts of the story that have been forgotten. Reverse roles and let the child tell you an incomplete version of the same story. Finish by telling the entire story with adequate detail. Audio record or videotape the story to share with parents and teachers.
Description	▶ Play "Twenty Questions" by putting a mystery object in a bag or box. The child should select the first object so that the clinician can model useful questions. Take turns asking questions for additional objects. Invite classmates to play the game so that they can also model questions. ▶ Describe the emotions displayed by children in photographs or stories. Encourage the child to describe situations when he has had similar feelings. ▶ Practice describing key attributes of a person (use career photos, family photos, or photos of school personnel), an object, or an action. Focus on telling the most salient characteristics of the item so that fewer clues are needed before the item is identified.
Explanation	▶ Explain why something happened to you or a family member through a personal story (e.g., Your son dropped his calculator and broke it because he was rushing to get to practice). Ask the child to share recent difficult situations and their causes (e.g., bike accident, missed assignment). ▶ Discuss how the child would explain a difficult situation (e.g., why you don't have lunch money today) to a friend using informal language and to an adult using more formal language. Role-play a variety of situations and persons.

continued on next page

Table 8.5. Examples of Activities to Improve the Use of Communication Functions, *continued*	
Explanation, *continued*	▶ Discuss basic science concepts from the child's classroom. Possible topics include seasons, the effects of temperature on water, and the habitats of various kinds of animals (e.g., birds, amphibians, reptiles). Have the child develop an illustrated oral report for classmates or younger children.
Instruction-Giving	▶ Before playing a familiar board game, review the instructions in the instruction booklet. Ask the child to tell you the directions again while you write them down. Compare the child's list to the official instructions. ▶ Arrange for the child to teach a familiar game to younger children. ▶ Introduce a new board game and teach the child to play it. Have the child explain the rules before playing it with classmates.
Persuasion	▶ Discuss a situation in which you had to convince someone of something important (e.g., getting your daughter to walk the dog after school). Be sure to model your thought processes and the other person's perspective. Ask the child to discuss similar situations. ▶ Ask the child to think of things he wants (e.g., more allowance, his own room, a pet) and then make a list of points to convince his parents. Role-play the situation with each of you taking turns as the parent and the child. ▶ Have the child think of a school situation that needs to be changed (e.g., being allowed to join in the soccer game on the playground). Discuss how to persuade others to make a change. Role-play and reflect on additional ways to persuade others.

In addition to developing communication skills, a conversation-based approach provides abundant opportunities to enhance listening, speech, and language skills in meaningful contexts. Children are actually participating in synthetic auditory training activities every time they listen to a clinician's stories, answer a question, or interact with other children in the group. Similarly, the correct production of speech targets, while not a requisite for a conversation, can be easily reinforced and encouraged so that generalization to conversational speech occurs. Focused conversations, in which a particular language construction is modeled and obligated frequently, can reinforce both conversational and linguistic abilities. For example, by imagining transportation in the year 2050, children are obligated to make sentences that contain future-tense verbs (see Kretschmer and Kretschmer 1988 and the Suggested Reading list on page 159 for more conversation-based intervention ideas). In short, conversations provide a vehicle for addressing listening, language, and speech needs in an integrated and personally meaningful way.

Literacy, Language, and Communication: Intertwined Skills

Implementing a communication-based approach requires that the child be given "authentic, yet important, communication problems that he might face on a regular basis" (Kretschmer 1997, p. 379). For many children with hearing loss, reading comprehension difficulties pose authentic communication problems daily. Thus, literacy activities provide a rich context for conversations and communication intervention. There are a multitude of approaches to developing literacy skills in children with hearing loss (see Luetke-Stahlman and Luckner 1991, Schirmer and Williams 2003 for reviews). However, the remainder of this section will focus on two methods that are well-aligned with the principles of communication-based language intervention: interactive storytelling and the Pearson model for improving reading comprehension (Pearson 1985).

Interactive Storytelling. The value of reading stories to children is universally acknowledged. Young children learn a great deal about language, reading behaviors (e.g., top to bottom, page by page), story organization (e.g., conflict and resolution), and psychology (e.g., human nature and morality) by listening to adults read. Rich communication opportunities arise as story reading and conversations are woven together through a process known as Interactive Storytelling (IS). Story readers use the following strategies when using IS to enhance literacy in young children with hearing loss (adapted from Kretschmer 1997, Schirmer and Williams 2003).

▶ The story is read aloud using an expressive style and the children's mode of communication.

▶ The reader frequently connects events in the text to the children's world knowledge and personal experiences.

▶ The reader explains new vocabulary, concepts, and figures of speech as they are encountered. Unfamiliar words are explained with reference to children's established vocabularies.

▶ The reader asks questions to see if the children understand key points in the story and responds to answers in a non-judgmental way.

▶ The reader makes inferences aloud about future events in the story and points out clues (both in the text and pictures) that helped her make these deductions.

Interactive storytelling has been shown to lead to increased engagement during reading activities, and improved fingerspelling, story retelling, and word recognition in preschool and early elementary school children (Andrews 1988, Andrews and Mason 1986a and 1986b, Williams and McClean 1997, cited in Schirmer and Williams 2003). These gains suggest that language, communication, prereading, and metacognitive abilities are enhanced as children participate in interactive storytelling activities. In addition, this approach has the potential to increase academic achievement when stories are selected from the classroom curriculum.

Pearson's Approach to Improving Reading Comprehension. Children's literature and instructional textbooks provide authentic contexts for communication and language intervention. Children's literature stimulates the imagination and exposes children to the beliefs, values, and customs of their society and other cultures. For clinical purposes, it also provides models of dialogues and organizational patterns that are important for holding conversations and narrating events. Similarly, textbooks supply information and instruction for a wide range of subjects, including science, language arts, social studies, and math. School-age children are well aware of the importance of textbook content and usually desire to understand it as well as their peers. Problems arise, however, when children lack the language skills and cognitive strategies needed to understand fully what they read.

It has long been known that reading is a difficult process for children who have hearing impairments. Karchmer and Mitchell (2003, p. 27) recently summarized their review of studies of reading achievement in this population by noting, "the average performance on tests of reading comprehension for deaf and hard-of-hearing children is roughly six grade equivalents lower than their hearing peers at age 15." Although children with CIs have relatively greater hearing acuity than deaf children who use hearing aids, their language deficits can, nonetheless, interfere with the attainment of age-level reading skills. The following section proposes a model for addressing children's communication and reading comprehension needs in an integrated way.

Pearson and colleagues (Pearson 1985, Pearson and Gallagher 1983) have proposed a model for improving reading comprehension that incorporates several key components of communication-based intervention: the use of conversations, an emphasis on the child's ability to apply knowledge, and overt modeling of thought processes by the teacher/clinician. When applied to classroom reading materials (i.e., classroom-selected stories or textbook assignments), the Pearson model has the potential to improve academic as well as communication skills. Here are the basic steps for implementing this approach (adapted from Pearson 1985).

Step 1: Before reading

▶ Introduce the selected reading materials by:

- Relating aspects of the story/textbook assignment to the child's prior knowledge

- Highlighting new vocabulary words and connecting them to words the child already knows

- Making predictions about the story with the child

Step 2: While reading the material together

▶ Fill in gaps in the child's knowledge as needed

▶ Discuss related experiences that the child may have

▶ Make predictions about what will happen

▶ Link unfamiliar concepts to the child's experiences and knowledge

▶ Model your thought process aloud

Step 3. After finishing the desired amount of text

▶ *Ask questions.* The clinician composes a set of questions about the reading passage before meeting with the child. The types of questions will depend on the child's language abilities (examples are provided on page 157 in a section on question selection). Then complete the following steps for each question.

▶ *Provide answers.* The question is answered aloud.

▶ *Find proof.* The answerer then finds the lines of text that support or prove the given answer.

▶ *Explain.* The answerer tells how he knows that the answer is correct or incorrect based on the proof he found.

Step 4: After a story or textbook assignment has been completed

▶ Discuss the most salient aspects of the story, the moral, the unexpected events, or the most important concepts learned.

▶ Discuss the frameworks of the story (e.g., character, setting, and plot) or the organization of the textbook chapter.

▶ Involve the child in synthesizing activities such as dramatizing; summarizing; creating new, but similar stories; and parodies.

▶ Illustrate textbook topics through drawings and collages, or summarize the material with a computer slide show. Develop short presentations for peers or younger students.

The length of the reading passage for each session will be based on the child's age, attention, and reading abilities. Some children may be able to read, answer questions, and discuss several pages at a time. Others may need smaller chunks of material at first, and so the tasks in Step 3 would be completed after a paragraph or two. In situations where the child has substantial reading difficulties, the clinician may decide to read the entire passage aloud or take turns reading portions of the passage with the student.

A schedule for the question-answer activities can be found in Table 8.6. This schedule is organized in weekly modules. The clinician models the processes of reading comprehension during the first week and then gradually increases student responsibilities in subsequent weeks.

Table 8.6. Schedule for Implementing Practice in Reading Comprehension (Pearson 1985) (T= teacher/clinician, S = student)				
	Asks Q	**Answers**	**Finds Proof**	**Explains**
Week 1	T	T	T	T
Week 2	T	S	T	T
Week 3	T	S	S	T
Week 4	T	S	S	S

As this schedule shows, the Pearson model provides scaffolding for children to learn how to comprehend what they read. Instruction gradually changes from total reliance on teacher modeling to students completing the three main tasks. During the first week, the teacher asks questions, gives oral answers, shows the student lines of text that verify the answer (finds proof), and explains how she knows the answer is correct. Students answer questions during week 2, answer and find proof in week 3, and complete all tasks except for asking the questions during week 4. Although the teacher usually develops the list of questions, it may be beneficial to have students compose additional questions as well. Adjustments in the amount of time per level are also possible. For example, clinicians may wish to emphasize a given step for more than one week.

Selecting Questions. Choosing appropriate questions is basic to improving reading comprehension—especially for children with language deficits. Asking questions that are "over the head" of a child will be ineffective and can be frustrating. In contrast, over-reliance on factual questions can be dull and lead to literal interpretations, with little or no understanding of non-literal meanings. Bloom's Taxonomy (Bloom 1956, see Table 8.7) is a hierarchy of understanding that can be useful in controlling the linguistic and cognitive difficulty of reading comprehension questions.

For children who have very limited question-answering ability, questions from Levels 1 and 2 may be a good starting place. That is, clinicians may wish to emphasize "wh" and other factual questions until they are sure the child understands the meanings of these forms. Questions from Levels 2 – 6 should not be ignored, however, especially if they are important for understanding a story or passage. In these cases, the clinician will want to model the thought processes that she used to make a prediction or understand important aspects of the story (e.g., a character's motivation) rather than requiring children to answer higher-level questions. For children with relatively better language and reading abilities, a greater emphasis on questions from Levels 4 – 6 can stimulate higher-level thinking and provide practice in problem-solving and persuasion. In general, a mix of questions that address the factual, inferential, and the non-literal aspects of the story or textbook passage is suggested. The six levels of Bloom's Taxonomy and examples of corresponding questions are presented in Table 8.7.

Table 8.7. Bloom's Taxonomy (1956) and Examples of Corresponding Questions

Level 1 questions call for factual understanding. Because they are used frequently and there are a considerable number of types, no examples are provided. Question examples for Levels 2- 6 are based on the novel *To Kill a Mockingbird* by Harper Lee (1960).

Level 1. Knowledge Remembering, Recognizing, Recalling	Who, What, When, Where, Did, Do, Can, Is, Are, Was, Were questions
Level 2. Comprehension Interpreting, Paraphrasing, Organizing	What three things made you suspicious of Bob Ewell? Which people were not friendly to Scout?
Level 3. Application Problem solving, Using facts to infer, Recognizing relationships	What choices did Jem and Scout have? Why is the mockingbird important? How did Atticus prove that Tom Robinson was not guilty?
Level 4. Analysis Classify Compare/contrast Identify parts	Why didn't Boo Radley leave his house? Which people acted prejudiced? Which acted fairly? How was Boo Radley like a mockingbird?
Level 5. Synthesis Combine ideas for new perspective, Make inferences, Alternative outcomes	What might have happened if ___? What could Scout have done instead of hiding? What would you have done if ___?
Level 6. Evaluation Make a value decision, Rank priorities, Justify an opinion	If you were the judge at Bob Ewell's trial, what punishment would you have given? Why do you think that would be fair?

Conclusion

Children with CIs have many intertwined needs as they strive to match the social and academic skills achieved by their peers. This chapter has provided frameworks for identifying those needs and addressing them in an integrated way. Working closely together, parents, clinicians, and teachers can develop practical, individualized plans to help children reach their full potentials as communicators, students, and citizens. The next chapter provides suggestions for ensuring that listening conditions are optimized throughout the school day: a task that also requires on-going collaboration among these stakeholders.

Suggested Reading

▶ *Blueprint for Developing Conversational Competence: A Planning / Instructional Model with Detailed Scenarios*
Stone, P. (1988)
A.G. Bell Association

▶ *Counseling Children with Hearing Impairment and Their Families*
English, K. M. (2002)
Allyn and Bacon

▶ *Language and Literacy Development in Children Who Are Deaf*
Schirmer, B. R. (1994)
Merrill Publishing

▶ *Let's Converse! A How-To Guide to Develop and Expand the Conversational Skills of Children and Teenagers Who Are Hearing Impaired*
Tye-Murray, N. (1994)
A.G. Bell Association

▶ *Literacy Learning for Children Who Are Deaf or Hard of Hearing*
Robertson, L. (2000)
A.G. Bell Association

References

Andrews, J. F. (1988a). Deaf children's acquisition of prereading skills using the reciprocal teaching procedure. *Exceptional Children*, 54, 349-355.

Andrews, J. F. and Mason, J. (1986a). Childhood deafness and the acquisition of print concepts. In D. Yaden and S. Templeton (Eds.), *Metalinguistic awareness and beginning literacy: Conceptualizing what it means to read and write* (pp. 277-290). Portsmouth, NH: Heinemann.

Andrews, J. F. and Mason, J. (1986b). How do deaf children learn about prereading? *American Annals of the Deaf*, 131, 210-217.

Barrett, M., Huisingh, R., Bowers, L., LoGiudice, C., Orman, J. (1992). *The listening test*. East Moline, IL: LinguiSystems, Inc.

Blamey, P. J. and Alcantara, J. I. (1994). Research in auditory training. *Journal of the Academy of Rehabilitative Audiology*, 27 (Suppl.), 161-192.

Blamey, P. J., Sarant, J. Z., Paatsch, L. E., Barry, J. G., Bow, C. P., Wales, R. J., et al. (2001). Relationships among speech perception, production, language, hearing loss, and age in children with impaired hearing. *Journal of Speech, Language, & Hearing Research*, 44(2), 264-285.

Bliele, K. M. (1995). *Manual of articulation and phonological disorders: Infancy through adulthood*. Clifton Park, NY: Delmar Learning.

Bloom, B. (1956). *Taxonomy of educational objectives: The classification of educational goals: Handbook 1: Cognitive domain*. New York: Longmans, Green, and Co.

Bowers, L., Huisingh, R., LoGiudice, C., and Orman, J. (2002). *Test of semantic skills–primary (TOSS–P)*. East Moline, IL: LinguiSystems, Inc.

Bowers, L., Huisingh, R., LoGiudice, C., and Orman, J. (2004). *Test of semantic skills–intermediate (TOSS–I)*. East Moline, IL: LinguiSystems, Inc.

Conner, C., Heiber, S., Arts, H., and Zwolan, T. A. (2000). Speech, vocabulary and the education of children using cochlear implants: Oral or total communication? *Journal of Speech-Language and Hearing Research*, 43, 1185-1204.

DiSimoni, F. (1978). *The token test for children*. Austin, TX: Pro-Ed.

160

References, *continued*

Ertmer, D. J. (2001). Emergence of a vowel system in a young cochlear implant recipient. *Journal of Speech-Language and Hearing Research*, 44, 803-813.

Ertmer, D. J. (2002). Auditory training for school-age children with cochlear implants: Addressing speech perception and oral communication needs. *Perspectives on Hearing and Hearing Disorders in Childhood*, 12, 29-32.

Ertmer, D. J. (2003). *Contrasts for auditory and speech training (CAST)*. East Moline, IL: LinguiSystems, Inc.

Ertmer, D. J., Leonard, J. S., and Pachuilo, M. L. (2002). Communication intervention for children with cochlear implants: Two case studies. *Language, Speech, and Hearing Services in Schools*, 33(3), 205-217.

Goldman, R. and Fristoe, M. (2000). *Goldman-Fristoe test of articulation-2*. Circle Pines, MN: American Guidance Services.

Greenberg, M. (1993, October). Family communication and coping: Developmental issues in promoting social competence. Paper presented at the Eighth Annual Conference on Issues in Language and Deafness, Boys Town National Research Hospital, Omaha, NE.

Health insurance portability and accountability act of 1996. Public Law 104-191.

Karcher, M. A. and Mitchell, R. E. (2003). Demographic and achievement characteristics of deaf and hard-of-hearing students. In M. Marschark and P. E. Spencer (Eds.), *Oxford handbook of deaf studies, language, and education*, (pp. 21-37). Oxford: Oxford University Press.

Khan, L. and Lewis, N. (2002). *Khan-Lewis phonological assessment-2*. Circle Pines, MN: American Guidance Services.

Kretschmer, R. (1997). Issues in the development of school and interpersonal discourse for children who have hearing loss. *Language, Speech, and Hearing Services in Schools*, 28, 374-383.

Kretschmer, R. and Kretschmer, L. (Eds.). (1988). Communication assessment of hearing impaired children: From conversation to classroom (Monograph). *The Journal of the Academy of Rehabilitative Audiology*, 21.

Lee, H. (1960). *To kill a mockingbird*. Philadelphia: Lippincott Williams & Wilkins, Inc.

Lehiste, I. (1970). *Suprasegmentals*. Cambridge, MA: MIT Press.

References, *continued*

Ling, D. (1976). *Speech and the hearing-impaired child: Theory and practice.* Washington, D.C: A.G. Bell Association.

Ling, D. (1989). *Foundations of spoken language development.* Washington, D.C.: A.G. Bell Association.

Lowe, R. (2000). *Assessing the link between phonology and articulation-revised (ALPHA–R).* Mifflinville, PA: Speech and Language Resources.

Luetke-Stahlman, B. and Luckner, J. (1991). *Effectively educating students with hearing impairments.* New York: Longman.

Miller, J. F. and Paul, R. (1995). *The clinical assessment of language comprehension.* Baltimore: Paul H. Brookes Publishing, Inc.

Moog, J. S. and Geers, A. E. (1990). *Early speech perception test for profoundly hearing-impaired children.* St. Louis: Central Institute for the Deaf.

Niparko, J., Cheng, A. and Francis, H. (2000). Outcomes of cochlear implantation: Assessment of quality of life impact and evaluation of the benefits of the cochlear implant in relation to costs. In J. Niparko, K. I. Kirk, N. Mellon, A. Robbins, D. Tucci, and B. Wilson (Eds.), *Cochlear implants: Principles and practices* (pp. 269-290*).* Philadelphia: Lippincott Williams & Wilkins, Inc..

Pearson, P. D. (1985). Changing the face of reading comprehension instruction. *The Reading Teacher,* 724 -738.

Pearson, P. D. and Gallagher, M. C. (1983). The instruction of reading comprehension. *Contemporary Educational Psychology,* 8, 317-344.

Robbins, A. M. (1994). *A critical evaluation of rehabilitation techniques.* Paper presented at the Fifth Symposium on Cochlear Implants in Children, New York.

Schirmer, B. R. and Williams, C. (2003). Approaches to Reading Instruction. In M. Marschark and P. Spencer (Eds.), *Oxford handbook of deaf studies, language, and education* (pp. 110 - 122). Oxford: Oxford University Press.

Stoel-Gammon, C. and Herrington, P. B. (1990). Vowel systems of normally developing and phonologically disordered children. *Clinical Linguistics and Phonetics,* 4, 145-160.

References, *continued*

Tye-Murray, N. and Kirk, K. (1993). Vowel and diphthong production by young users of cochlear implants and the relationship between the Phonetic Level Evaluation and spontaneous speech. *Journal of Speech and Hearing Research*, 36, 488-502.

Wilkes, E. M. (1999). *Cottage acquisition scales for listening, language, and speech.* San Antonio, TX: Sunshine Cottage.

Williams, C. and McClean, M. (1997). Young deaf children's response to picture book reading in a preschool setting. *Research in the Teaching of English*, 31, 337-366.

Wood, D. and Wood, H. (1997). Communicating with children who are deaf: Pitfalls and possibilities. *Language Speech and Hearing Services in the Schools*, 28, 348-354.

Yoshinaga-Itano, C. and Downey, D. M. (1986). A hearing-impaired child's acquisition of schemata: Something's missing. *Topics in Language Disorders*, 7, 45-57.

Optimizing Listening in the School Environment

9

Classrooms can be very difficult environments for listening and learning. Internal room noises (e.g., the hum of florescent lighting, the screech of sliding chairs, and the drone of ventilation systems) and external commotion (e.g., hallway noise) are frequently present at unacceptable levels in schools. Excessive noise can disrupt learning for students who have normal hearing, and it is especially detrimental for children with hearing problems (Nelson and Soli 2000). Speech-language pathologists, educational audiologists,

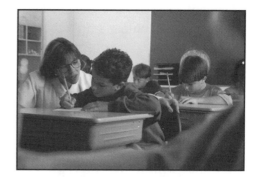

and teachers of children with hearing loss must be actively involved in improving school listening conditions if children with cochlear implants (CIs) are to be successful auditory learners in the classroom. This chapter provides the reader with necessary information for this undertaking. Four main topics are covered: the acoustic characteristics of classrooms, ways to reduce classroom noise levels, practical accommodations to improve auditory comprehension, and technologies that improve the quality of the speech signal before it reaches the listener.

Classroom Acoustics

Two measurements are used to describe classroom acoustics: Signal-to-Noise Ratio (SNR) and Reverberation Time (RT). Simply put, *SNR* is calculated as the difference in intensity between the signal of interest (e.g., the teacher's voice) and background noise. For example, if the intensity of a teacher's voice is measured at 65 dB SPL and the ambient noise level at 50 dB SPL, then the SNR is +15 decibels. Conversely, if the signal is less intense than the background noise (e.g., 55 and 80 dB SPL, respectively), a negative SNR exists (i.e., -25 dB SPL). A minimum SNR of +15 dB has been recommended for classrooms with children who have hearing losses (Crandell and Smaldino 2001).

In addition to the detrimental effects of noise, SNR becomes poorer as the distance between talker and the listener increases. For example, if the teacher's voice is 65 dB at the front of the classroom and an air conditioner produces a 50 dB "hum" in the back of the room, SNR will be well below the recommended level for children in the middle and back of the room. Unfortunately, the combination of high noise levels found in many unoccupied classrooms (Knecht et al. 2002) and the sounds produced during normal classroom activities can make it difficult to maintain the recommended SNR level.

Reverberation Time refers to the amount of time it takes for a steady-state signal to decrease from its peak intensity level by 60 dB. Some speech sounds (primarily vowels) can remain relatively intense after they are reflected off of hard surfaces such as walls and windows. Problems arise as these "echoes" overlap with the more recent, non-reflected speech signal and interfere with students' comprehension of spoken messages. Given this potential difficulty, it has been recommended that classroom RTs not exceed 0.4 seconds in environments where individuals with hearing losses are present (Crandell and Smaldino 2001). Current estimates suggest that only about a quarter of the classrooms in the U.S. meet this criteria (Crandell and Smaldino 1995).

Reducing Classroom Noise Levels

Measurements of SNR and RT are complex and require sophisticated instrumentation. A trained professional (e.g., audiologist, architect, engineer) is needed to identify and measure sources of excessive noise and estimate reverberation times. There are, however, a number of relatively simple modifications that can make classrooms less noisy and reverberant (see Table 9.1 on page 166). Most of these involve covering hard surfaces with sound-absorbing materials and muffling persistent sources of noise as much as possible.

Table 9.1: Suggestions for Reducing Classroom Noise and Reverberation

▶ "Tune-up" heating and cooling systems to make them run quietly.

▶ Keep hallway doors closed to limit external noise.

▶ Close windows whenever outside activities become noisy.

▶ Cover large windows with curtains to reduce reverberation.

▶ Apply sound-absorbing panels to walls to reduce reverberation.

▶ Make instructional "quiet zones" by placing barrier walls (similar to those used to form office cubicles) around a few tables or desks.

▶ Carpet the floor if possible.

▶ Place felt pads on the feet of chairs and desks if the floor cannot be carpeted.

▶ Repair light fixtures that "hum" or "buzz" excessively.

Enhancing Auditory Comprehension

Although the suggestions in Table 9.1 will reduce noise and reverberation, classrooms full of children are, by nature, noisy places. Despite improved room acoustics, the teacher's voice may be frequently masked by the ambient sounds and speech that students produce. To succeed in a regular classroom, children with CIs must be able to distinguish between noise and relevant information (i.e., oral instructions, peer communication). This task can require considerable energy whenever classroom SNRs are below recommended levels, and may lead to fatigue and learning difficulties when poor listening conditions are persistent. Fortunately, there are easy-to-implement teacher accommodations that can make auditory comprehension easier for children with CIs. Examples of these are presented in Table 9.2.

Table 9.2: Accommodations to Improve Listening Conditions and Auditory Comprehension	
Positional Accommodations	• Preferential seating; seat the student close to the teacher with the CI microphone on the side nearest the teacher and toward as many classmates as possible. • Seat the child away from sources of noise, including heating and cooling units, hallway doors, and windows near streets or playgrounds. • Seat the child across from the teacher during small group activities. • Arrange preferential positioning in art, gym, music classes, and other special activities (e.g., assemblies).
Visual Accommodations	• Write daily and weekly schedules and assignments on chalk/white board. • Have students keep an assignment notebook. • Use drawings and diagrams to supplement spoken explanations of new concepts. • Be sure the child can see the chalk/white board well. • Give instructions from a well-lit location so speechreading cues can be seen easily.
Instructional Accommodations	• Get the child's attention before giving directions; insist on eye-contact throughout the message. • Speak directly to the child as often as possible when giving instructions. • Avoid talking when your back is turned to the child. • Speak slightly louder and more slowly than normal while articulating clearly. • Rephrase (rather than repeat) your message when the child appears puzzled. • Allow extra time for a response when asking questions. • Do not assume that the child understands new information. Check for comprehension by asking the child to repeat or rephrase what was said. • Repeat other students' questions and comments aloud so the child can hear them better. • Encourage the child to ask questions and ask for clarification.
Other Possible Accommodations	• Assign a classmate to be a note taker during lectures. • Provide an oral or sign interpreter as needed. • Select a responsible classmate to be a "listening buddy." This student will share information and answer any questions about classroom activities. Allow the CI user to ask the listening buddy questions as often as necessary. • Adjust the amount of material on tests and/or the amount of time allowed for testing according to the child's needs.

Specific accommodations for children with CIs should be selected during multi-disciplinary case conferences and included in IEPs. Because accommodations can be beneficial during most school activities, chosen strategies should be used in special classes (e.g., gym, art, and music) and during assemblies, as well as in the regular classroom. It is also important to encourage children with CIs to take responsibility for understanding classroom communication. Reliance on accommodations should be decreased gradually as the student becomes a conscientious listener. Clinicians should monitor the use of accommodations and offer suggestions for adding new strategies and discarding unnecessary ones. Although accommodations can improve auditory comprehension in noisy environments, children with CIs are also likely to benefit from using assistive listening technology.

Assistive Listening Devices

Assistive Listening Devices (ALDs) overcome noise, excessive reverberation, and distance by placing a microphone close to the talker's mouth and transmitting an enhanced speech signal to the listener. Children are able to understand this improved signal more easily because it has a high SNR. Two main types of ALDs are used by children with cochlear implants in regular school settings: FM and infrared systems.

As the name indicates, wireless FM systems use radio waves to transmit the teacher's voice to the child's receiver unit without a connecting cable. There are three main kinds of wireless FM systems: personal, desktop, and classroom amplification. Each of these systems has a teacher-worn microphone-transmitter unit (See Figure 9.1) and a signal receiver unit. The receivers convey the enhanced signal to the listener in several different ways.

Personal FM systems connect an FM receiver unit to the individual's implant speech processor via adapter cables (sometimes called "patch cords"), direct coupling (connecting the receiver to the CI without a cable), or a telecoil (an optional setting on some CIs that allows the implant to process electromagnetic signals) depending on the features of the implant and the connection chosen by

Figure 9.1: Teacher Wearing an ALD Mic-Transmitter Unit

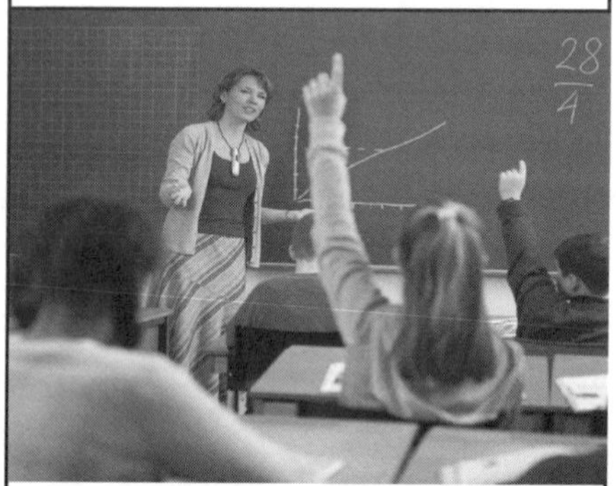

(Courtesy of Phonic Ear Corporation)

the audiologist. Figure 9.2 shows an ear-level FM receiver unit that can be coupled directly to some Advanced Bionics and MED-EL implant systems. Personal FM systems can be used with a single child or a group of children wearing receivers that are set to the same FM frequency.

FM desktop systems consist of small, lightweight receiver-loudspeaker units that pick up the signal from the teacher's transmitter, amplify it, and project it acoustically from close range. Figure 9.3 shows a complete desktop system including a head-worn microphone, transmitter (small, gray box), and mini receiver-loudspeaker unit. This system can easily be transported from room to room by the user.

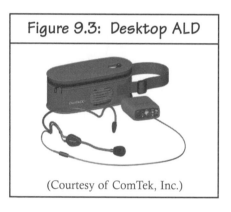

Figure 9.2: The Lexis FM Receiver

(Courtesy of Phonic Ear Corporation)

FM classroom amplification systems use multiple, wall- or ceiling-mounted loudspeakers to present the teacher's voice at a constant loudness level throughout the room. All students in the classroom (those with normal hearing and those with hearing losses) benefit from the much-improved SNR that this type of system provides (Crandell et al. 1995). FM classroom amplification systems consist of a microphone-transmitter unit, a receiver, an amplifier, and a set of loudspeakers.

Figure 9.3: Desktop ALD

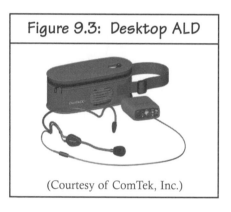

(Courtesy of ComTek, Inc.)

Recent improvements in technology have also made *infrared ALD systems* viable options for classroom amplification. Infrared systems convert sound into light energy and transmit an enhanced speech signal to the listener via an invisible infrared carrier beam. A receiver-amplifier unit picks up this signal, increases its power, and conveys it to loudspeakers that project it acoustically from various positions around the classroom. The components of an infrared classroom amplification system can be seen in Figure 9.4.

Figure 9.4: Telex IR System

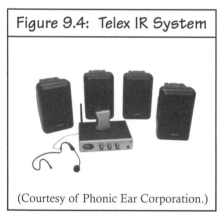

(Courtesy of Phonic Ear Corporation.)

Resources that describe the advantages and disadvantages of FM, infrared, and other ALD technologies can be found in the Suggested Reading list on page 171.

Selecting and fitting an ALD system requires close collaboration between audiologists, implant professionals, and classroom teachers. Daily listening checks are also needed to ensure that both the ALD and the implant are functioning properly. Web sites for each implant manufacturer offer information regarding these tasks.

Summary

The combined use of environmental modifications, student accommodations, and ALDs can greatly improve listening and learning conditions in noisy environments. If children with CIs are to reach their social and academic potentials, speech-language pathologists, audiologists, and teachers of children with hearing loss must be leaders in providing and maintaining these services. The final chapter of this book continues to explore technological and educational issues by considering what the future may hold for children with hearing losses.

Suggested Reading

▶ *Assistive Devices for Persons with Hearing Impairment*
R. S. Tyler and D. J. Schum (Eds.) (1995)
Allyn and Bacon

▶ *Educational Audiology Handbook*
DeConde Johnson, C., Benson, P., and Seaton, J. (1997)
Singular Publishing Group

Internet Resources

▶ http://www.bionicear.com/support/betterliving/ald.asp
The Advanced Bionics Web site provides information about coupling FM
ALDs with various Clarion CIs, troubleshooting, and contact information
for ALD manufacturers.

▶ http://www.cochlearamericas.com/151.asp
The Cochlear Americas Web site contains information about CI compatible
ALDs, the use of telecoils, and techniques for using the telephone with an
implant.

▶ http://www.medel.com/ENG/US/20_Products/30_Accessories/
000_tempo_accessories.asp
Information for purchasing adapter cables for MED-EL cochlear implant
systems can be found on this Web page.

▶ http://clerccenter.gallaudet.edu/InfoToGo/418.html
A broad overview of assistive devices is presented on this Web site
developed at Gallaudet University.

▶ http://www.raisingdeafkids.org/help/tech/ald/faq.jsp
Answers to frequently asked questions about ALDs are presented at the
"Raising Deaf Kids" Web site.

References

Compton, C. L. (1995). Selecting what's best for the individual. In R. S. Tyler and D. J. Schum (Eds.), *Assistive devices for persons with hearing impairment* (pp. 224-250). Needham Heights, MD: Allyn & Bacon.

Crandell, C. and Smaldino, J. (1995). An update of classroom acoustics for children with hearing impairment. *Volta Review*, 97, 4-12.

Crandell, C. and Smaldino, J. (2001). Classroom acoustics for children with normal hearing and hearing impairment. *Language, Speech, and Hearing Services in Schools*, 31, 362-370.

Crandell, C., Smaldino, J., and Flexer, C. (1995). *Soundfield FM: Application theory and practical applications.* Singular Publishing Group: San Diego.

Knetch, H. A., Nelson, P. B., Whitelaw, G. M., and Feth, L. L. (2002). Background noise levels and reverberation times in unoccupied classrooms: Predictions and measurements. *American Journal of Audiology*, 11, 65.

Nelson, P. and Soli, S. (2000). Acoustic barriers to learning: Children at risk in every classroom. *Language, Speech, and Hearing Services in Schools*, 31, 356-361.

Future Developments in Technology and Intervention

10

Cochlear Implant Technology

In the rapidly changing field of cochlear implant technology, a look to the future must also include an appreciative glance to the recent past. Indeed, the last 20 years have produced many remarkable advancements that support contemporary and future developments. The following are a few of the areas in which significant improvements have been made.

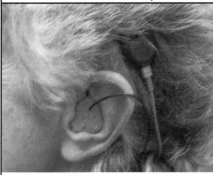

Figure 10.1: Hearing Aid Serving as a Preprocessor for a Cochlear Implant

(Used with permission from K. Chung)

Speech processing strategies. Advancements in speech processing have been aimed at making speech easier to understand. Contemporary strategies such as CIS, ACE, and n of m have been developed to help individuals at the lower end of the performance continuum achieve better outcomes (Wilson 2000).

Electrode array designs. Recent advances in technology have resulted in electrode arrays that permit single electrodes or groups of electrodes to stimulate the auditory nerve over relatively small areas. These more "focused" arrays allow for greater numbers of discrete channels of information while reducing the spread of electrical current.

MRI-compatible receiver-stimulators. The development of internal implant components that are unaffected by Magnetic Resonation Imaging (MRI) allows CI users to have access to this important medical technology.

Behind The Ear (BTE) cochlear implants. These relatively small units provide convenience, comfort, and cosmetic benefits for many implant users.

Penetrating auditory brainstem implants. These sensory aids are designed to improve hearing ability for individuals who have damage to the auditory nerve and cannot benefit from cochlear implantation.

Improved power source. Today's implant batteries provide energy for considerably longer periods of time than was possible in the early 1990s. Rechargeable batteries also have longer life spans.

Further evidence that the "future is now" can be seen in more recent cochlear implant developments. Investigations are currently underway to determine the feasibility and efficacy of a wide variety of technological improvements. The following is but a small sampling of the areas being explored.

Bilateral cochlear implants. Initial research findings suggest that adults who have two implants can localize sounds better than those with one (Van Hoesel et al. 2002, see Wilson 2003 for review). Speech perception in noise may also be enhanced by having two implants. The benefits of bilateral implantation for children are currently being examined.

The combined use of hearing aids and CIs in the same ear. Many hard-of-hearing individuals have high frequency hearing losses with usable residual hearing in the low- and mid-frequency ranges. Experiments are underway to determine whether it is feasible and effective to combine electrical stimulation via a shortened electrode array with conventional amplification (McDermott 2001, Wilson 2003).

Further improvements in electrode array designs. Manufacturers continue to refine electrode array designs, seeking ways to provide simultaneous electrode activation while decreasing interaction between channels. New arrays will increase the number of channels of information that are available to the listener and use power more efficiently (Wilson 2003).

Built-in FM receiver units. Hearing aids with internal FM receivers became available in the early 1990s. This combination of technologies allows children to more easily use their Assistive Listening Devices (ALDs) at home as well as at school. It is likely that children with CIs will soon benefit from the integration of these technologies.

Improved hearing under difficult listening conditions. Comprehending speech in noisy environments is the ultimate auditory challenge for CI and hearing aid users alike. Digital hearing aids use a variety of strategies to reduce the impact of background noise without affecting the quality of the speech signal. Efforts are underway to apply these strategies for the benefit of cochlear implant users (Chung et al. 2004; see Figure 10.1).

Spurred on by commercial competition, cochlear implant manufacturers are constantly seeking ways to improve or expand the uses of their products. The following is just a glimpse of some of the potential advancements in cochlear implant technology that may become reality.

The Source for Children with Cochlear Implants　　　175

Further reductions in the size of implant components. Reductions in the size of cochlear implants could lead to dramatic changes in surgical procedures and improved performance. For instance, the development of "in the ear" or "in the canal" CIs would permit access to the cochlea via the tympanic membrane and middle ear space. Such small devices would eliminate the need for an incision behind the ear and for drilling through the temporal bone, making implant surgery simpler and safer. Taking the miniaturization process one step further, the cochlear implants of the future may become so small that they could be housed in the middle ear space (Wilson 2000). Such a location would take advantage of the natural, speech-enhancing resonance characteristics of the outer ear, make re-implantation easier in the event of device failure, and have the cosmetic benefit of being practically invisible.

Stimulation of nerve cell growth. One of the most forward-thinking ideas in the field of CI technology goes beyond electrical stimulation of the auditory nerve. Although clinical trials have not begun, neuroscientists are considering the possibility of using cochlear implants to deliver chemicals called "growth factors" to the inner ear. Theoretically, growth factors could help to regrow or stimulate the development of new hair cells in Organ of Corti. If exploratory studies are successful, the CI of tomorrow could have two main functions: to stimulate the auditory nerve electrically and to act as a miniature pump to introduce chemicals for the revitalization of hearing structures (Holley 2003).

Intervention Issues

As mentioned in the Preface, cochlear implant technology alone will not enable individuals to reach their auditory-oral communication potentials in an efficient manner. Intensive communication intervention is needed to help children take full advantage of improved hearing ability. Just as engineers and designers seek to improve CI technology, so too, clinicians, researchers and educators must strive to increase the effectiveness of post-implantation intervention practices. There are several significant challenges in the latter area.

Factors that Influence Service Delivery

Children who receive cochlear implants require communication intervention services to optimize auditory-oral learning. Fortunately, in the U.S., these services are mandated from birth through 21 years of age. Thus, all children should have access to quality intervention programs. Several factors, however, can significantly impact the quality of communication intervention services for children with CIs. These include level of parental support, availability of specialized services, level of professional preparation, and administrative issues. Each of these factors must be addressed if current and future CI users are to take full advantage of improvements in implant technology.

Parental Support for Post-Implantation Services

Although most parents are very supportive of communication intervention services, some parents fail to take full advantage of these programs. The need for, and the value of, communication intervention is routinely emphasized during the implant candidacy process. Parental commitment to the intervention process, however, may not be apparent until after the child has received a CI. One way to assess commitment to follow-up services is to involve the family in an intervention program prior to making the implantation decision. Adequate commitment will be evident when services are well-attended and parents actively participate in intervention activities. Parental commitment to communication intervention should be assessed prior to making the decision to provide an implant.

Availability of the Specialized Services

Because hearing loss is a low incidence disability, children who live in rural and small town settings often have fewer educational and communication options than those who live in cities. As a result, they might not have access to an early interventionist with experience in hearing impairment or cochlear implants, are more likely to be placed in multi-categorical special education classrooms, and/or might have only one option for a mode of communication at school (e.g., total communication classroom). The lack of trained personnel and specialized curriculum for children with hearing loss can have serious consequences for communication development after implantation (Ertmer et al. 2002). Fortunately, some of these problems can be addressed as parents and local educators interact with state-supported outreach programs and use the child's CI team as a resource for intervention models and educational planning. Implant manufacturers also offer assistance to local educators. For example, Advanced Bionics, Inc. offers the "Tools for Schools" program to assist professionals in meeting the communication and academic needs of children with CIs. This resource can be found at *http://www.bionicear.com/support/betterliving/bea.asp.*

Professional Preparation

As mentioned in the Preface, many practicing SLPs, audiologists, and teachers of children with hearing loss have had little or no academic work or clinical training in the area of cochlear implants. Because the number of children with CIs is steadily increasing, there is a pressing need to disseminate information about CI technology and intervention methods to early interventionists and school-based practitioners. Similarly, students in the field of communication disorders should have access to courses in aural rehabilitation that include both cochlear implant technology and related intervention approaches. These challenges can be addressed through a combination of increased in-service training, clinical forums in professional journals (e.g., Ertmer 2002, Schery 2003), continuing education opportunities, Internet resources, teleconferences, the development of new university courses, and books with a clinical, as well as technical focus.

Administrative Issues

Even with proper training and prior experience, some clinicians may find that large caseloads affect the provision of adequate amounts of service to children with implants. As discussed in Chapters 6 – 8, children with CIs have broad communication deficits. Addressing the full range of their auditory, speech, language, and communication needs requires regular and intensive intervention. A recent large-scale study by Geers (2002) revealed that school-age children who were implanted by five years of age received an average of 80 – 90 minutes of communication intervention per week during their first four years of implant use. The substantial amount of time allotted for these children indicates that staffing teams viewed communication intervention as an IEP priority. Intervention programs that provide comparatively little treatment (e.g. 20-minute sessions, twice weekly) are not likely to help children develop their abilities efficiently. Effective intervention programs will also include designated times for consultation among the professionals who work with children with CIs.

Areas for Clinical Research

In general, the clinical methods proposed in this book are based on research in acoustic phonetics, theories of speech processing, research findings for children with communication disorders (especially those with hearing losses), and currently accepted practices for children with CIs. These methods must still be examined in a systematic way so that their effectiveness can be determined and improvements to clinical practices can be made. Research is also needed to further explain the effects of various within-child factors (e.g., intelligence, severity of hearing loss) and external factors (e.g., type of speech processing strategy, communication modality) on the development of listening, speech, language, and reading skills in very young implant recipients. These investigations take on increasing importance as clinicians attempt to prepare children for mainstream educational settings as efficiently as possible, and as CI developers refine implant technology to improve auditory comprehension for all users.

Conclusion

As the preceding paragraphs underscored, the field of cochlear implantation is rapidly changing. As a result, clinicians will be challenged to keep up with the latest advances in technology and intervention approaches in the years to come. It is hoped that *The Source for Children with Cochlear Implants* has provided readers with a foundation for understanding the special abilities and needs of children with CIs, as well as a thirst for additional knowledge in this exciting area.

References

Chung, K., Zeng, F. and Waltzman, S. (2004). Using hearing aid directional microphones and noise reduction algorithms to enhance cochlear implant performance. *Acoustics Research Letters Online*, 5(2), 56-61.

Ertmer, D. J. (Ed.). (2002). Challenges in optimizing oral communication in children with cochlear implants [Clinical Forum]. *Language, Speech, and Hearing Services in Schools*, 33(3).

Ertmer, D. J., Leonard, J. S., and Pachuilo, M. L. (2002). Communication intervention for children with cochlear implants: Two case studies. *Language, Speech and Hearing Services in the Schools*, 33(3), 205-217.

Geers, A. (2002). Factors affecting the development of speech, language, and literacy in children with early cochlear implantation. *Language, Speech and Hearing Services in the Schools*, 33, 172-183.

Holley, M. (2003). *Future for cochlear implants.* Retrieved October 19, 2004, from Defeating Deafness Web site, *www.defeatingdeafness.org*.

McDermott, H. (2001). *Current advances in cochlear implants.* Retrieved October 19, 2004, from Defeating Deafness Web site, *www.defeatingdeafness.org*.

Schery, T. (Ed.). (2003). Cochlear implants in children: Ideas for intervention. *Topics in Language Disorders*, 23(1).

Van Hoesel, R. M., Ramsden, R., and O'Driscoll, M. (2002). Sound direction identification, interaural time delay discrimination, and speech intelligibility advantages in noise for a bilateral cochlear implant user. *Ear and Hearing*, 23, 137-149.

Wilson, B. (2000). Cochlear implant technology. In J. Niparko, K. I. Kirk, N. Mellon, A. Robbins, D. Tucci, and B. Wilson (Eds.), *Cochlear implants: Principles & practices* (pp. 109-118). Philadelphia: Lippincott Williams and Wilkins, Inc.

Wilson, B. (2003). Cochlear implants: Some likely next steps. *Annual Review of Biomedical Engineering*, 5, 207-249.